EAT FOR ENERGY

C·R·E·A·T·I·O·N Health

LIFE GUIDE #8

For Individual Study and Small Group Use

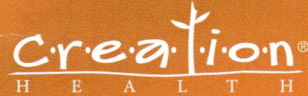

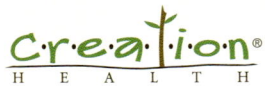

CREATION Health Life Guide #8
Copyright © MMXIII by Florida Hospital
Published by Florida Hospital Publishing
900 Winderley Place, Suite 1600
Maitland, Florida 32751

To Extend the Health and Healing Ministry of Christ

Publisher and Editor-in-Chief:	Todd Chobotar
Managing Editor:	David Biebel, DMin
Production:	Lillian Boyd
Promotion:	Laurel Prizigley
Copy Editor:	Pamela Nordberg
Author Photography:	Timothy Brown
Design:	Carter Design, Inc., Denver, CO
Peer Reviewers:	George Guthrie, MD; Karen Tilstra, PhD
	Sherri Flynt, MPH, RD, LD; Barbara Olsen, MACL
	Sabine Vatel, DMin; Andy McDonald, DMin; Tim Goff, MDiv
	Rick Szilagyi, DMin; Gerald Wasmer, MDiv
	Andre VanHeerden; Paul Campoli, MDiv

Publisher's Note: This book is not intended to replace a one-on-one relationship with a qualified healthcare professional, but as a sharing of knowledge and information from the research and experience of the author. You are advised and encouraged to consult with your healthcare professional in all matters relating to your health and the health of your family. The publisher and author disclaim any liability arising directly or indirectly from the use of this book.

The author assumes full responsibility for the accuracy of all facts and quotations as cited in this book. CREATION Health is a registered trademark of Florida Hospital. All rights reserved.

NOT TO BE REPRODUCED
No portion of this book may be reproduced, stored in a retrieval system, or transmitted in any form or by any means – electronic, mechanical, photocopy, recording, or any other – except for brief quotations in printed reviews, without the prior written permission of the publisher. All rights reserved.

Unless otherwise indicated, all Scripture quotations are taken from the Holy Bible, New Living Translation, copyright © 1996, 2004 by Tyndale House Publishers, Inc., Wheaton, Illinois 60189. All other Scripture references are from the following sources: The Holy Bible, New International Version (NIV), copyright © 1973, 1978, 1984 by Biblica, Inc. Used by permission of Zondervan. The Holy Bible, King James Version (KJV). The Holy Bible, New King James Version (NKJV), copyright © 1982 by Thomas Nelson, Inc. Good News Translation ® (Today's English Version, Second Edition) Copyright © 1992 American Bible Society. English Standard Version ® (ESV®), copyright © 2001 by Crossway, a publishing ministry of Good News Publishers. All Scriptures used by permission. All rights reserved.

For volume discounts please contact special sales at:
HealthProducts@FLHosp.org | 407-303-1929

Printed in the United States of America.
PR 14 13 12 11 10 9 8 7 6 5 4 3 2 1
ISBN: 978-0-9887406-6-2

For more life-changing resources visit:
FloridaHospitalPublishing.com
Healthy100Churches.org
CREATIONHealth.com
Healthy100.org

CONTENTS

Introduction – Welcome to CREATION Health	4
1. God's Amazing Gift	6
2. The Joy of Eating	18
3. The Good Stuff – Part A	30
4. The Good Stuff – Part B	42
5. Let's Go Shopping	56
6. Frugal and Fast	70
7. Feed Your Brain	82
8. Eating Together	94
About the Author	107
Notes	108
Resources	117

DOWNLOAD YOUR FREE LEADER RESOURCE

Are you a small group leader? We've created a special resource to help you lead an effective CREATION Health discussion group. Download at: **CREATIONHealth.com/LeaderResources**

WELCOME TO CREATION HEALTH

Congratulations on your choice to use this resource to improve your life! Whether you are new to the concept of CREATION Health or are a seasoned expert, this book was created for you. CREATION Health is a faith-based health and wellness program based on the Bible's Creation story. This book is part of a Life Guide series seeking to help you apply eight elegantly simple principles for living life to the full.

The letters of the CREATION acronym stand for:

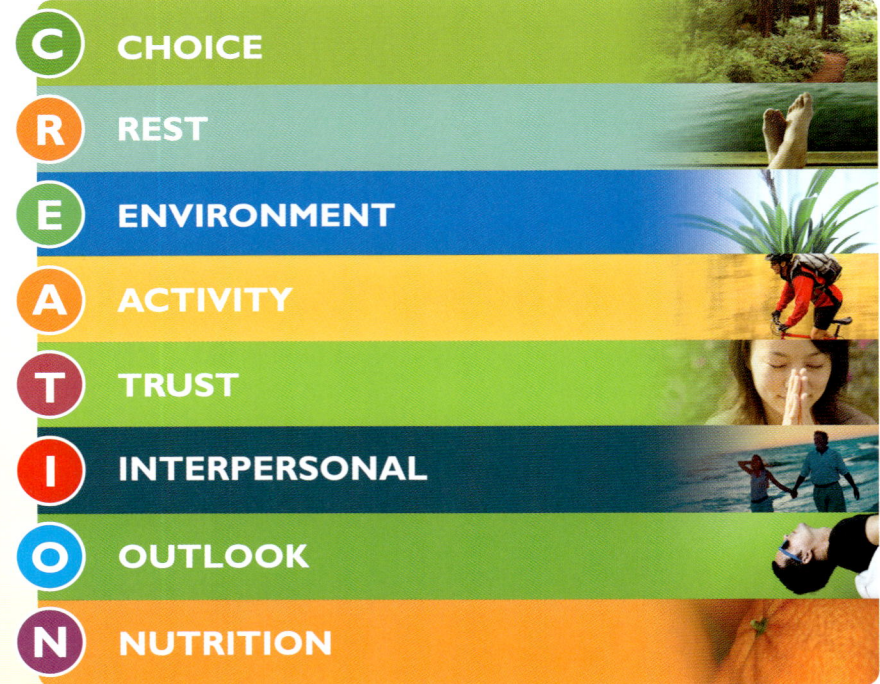

- **C** CHOICE
- **R** REST
- **E** ENVIRONMENT
- **A** ACTIVITY
- **T** TRUST
- **I** INTERPERSONAL
- **O** OUTLOOK
- **N** NUTRITION

In John 10:10 Jesus said, "I have come that they may have life, and have it to the full" (NIV). The Greek word used for life is "zoe," which means the absolute fullness of life…genuine life…a life that is active, satisfying, and filled with joy.

That is why CREATION Health takes a life-transforming approach to total person wellness – mentally, physically, spiritually, and socially – with the eight universal principles of health. Where did these principles come from?

The book of Genesis describes how God created the Earth and made a special garden called Eden as a home for his first two children, Adam and Eve. One of the first and finest gifts given to them was abundant health. By examining the Creation story we can learn much about feeling fit and living long, fulfilling lives today.

As you begin this journey toward an improved lifestyle, remember that full health is more than the absence of disease and its symptoms. It's a realization that God desires each of his children – people like you and me whom he loves and cares about – to have the best that this life can offer. It is trusting that your Creator has a plan for your life.

Is there any good parent who doesn't want the best for their child? No. So it makes sense that God would want his best for us. Naturally, human freedom of choice sometimes makes life messy, so not everything can or will be perfect as it once was. But that doesn't mean we shouldn't take a good look at the earliest records of humans found in the Bible to see if there is something special that can be gleaned.

This book – and the other seven in the Life Guide series – takes a deep dive into CREATION Health and translates the fundamental concepts into easy-to-follow steps. These guides include many questions designed to help you or your small group plumb the depths of every principle and learn strategies for integrating the things you learn into everyday life. As a result, you will discover that embracing the CREATION Health prescription can help restore health, happiness, balance, and joy to life.

The CREATION Health Lifestyle has a long, proven history of wellness and longevity – worldwide! People just like you are making a few simple changes in their lives and living longer, fuller lives. They are getting healthy, staying healthy, and are able to do the things they love, well into their later years. Now is the time to join them by transforming your habits into a healthy lifestyle.

If you would like to learn more about the many resources available, visit **CREATIONHealth.com**. If you would like to learn more about how to live to a Healthy 100, visit **Healthy100.org** or visit **Healthy100Churches.org**.

Welcome to CREATION Health,

Todd Chobotar
Publisher and Editor-in-Chief

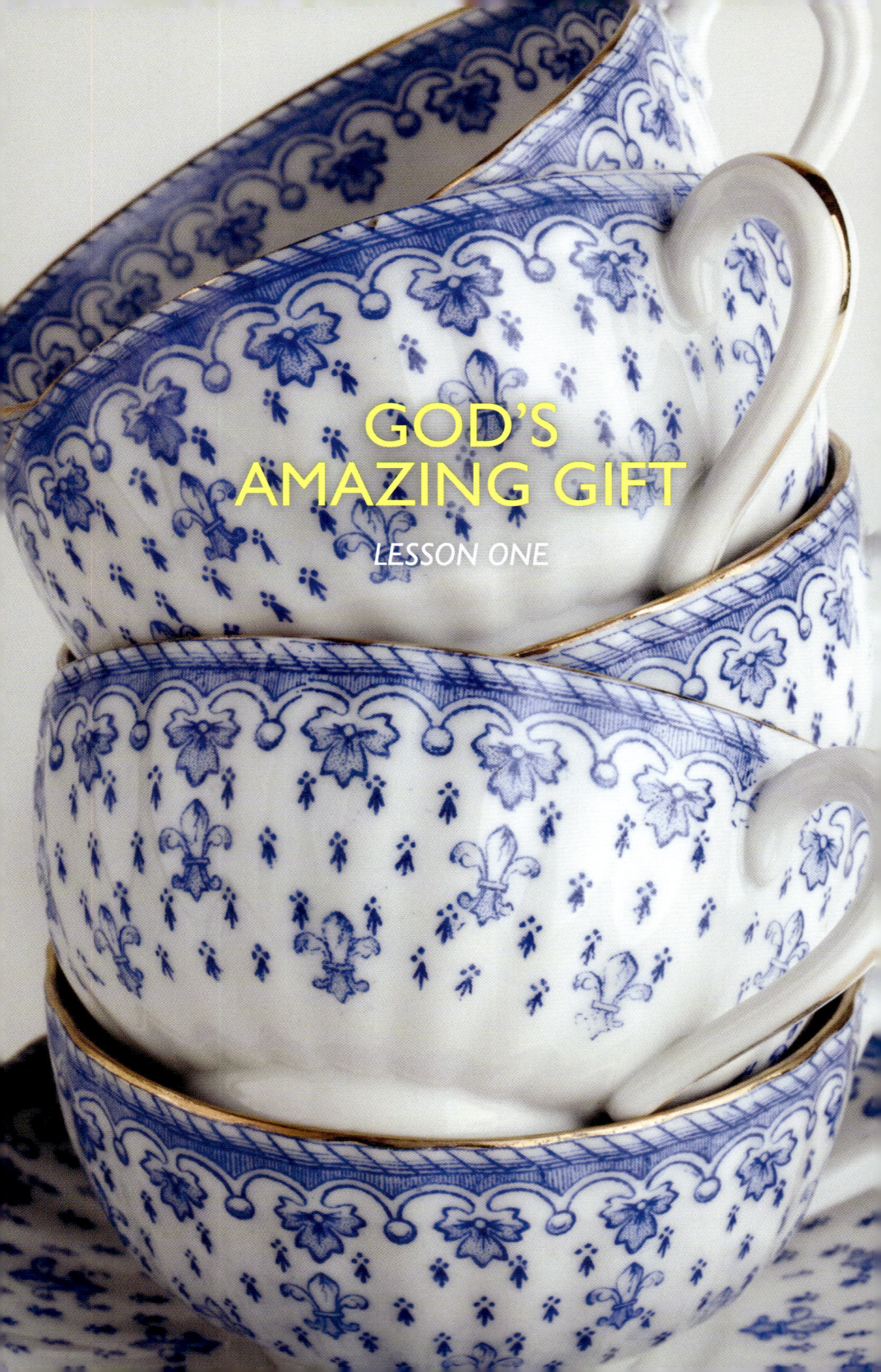

GOD'S AMAZING GIFT

LESSON ONE

WARM UP

Choose one or both questions to discuss (if in group setting) or write out your answers on a separate sheet (for individual use):

1. **What item from your childhood home would you like to have now?**[1]

   ....
   ....
   ....
   ....
   ....

2. **What has been your greatest source of joy in the last five years?**[2]

   ....
   ....
   ....
   ....
   ....
   ....

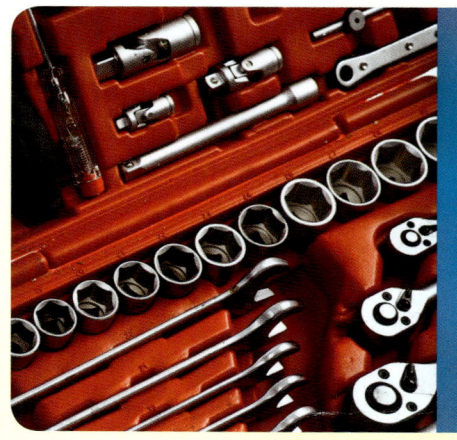

"A man too busy to take care of his health is like a mechanic too busy to take care of his tools."

SPANISH PROVERB

DISCOVERY

I was asked to give a devotional talk to a small group of a dozen people, and I used a tea cup as an illustration. It was white with dark blue designs that included tiny flowers hanging from thin, twisting vines, a couple of bridges arching over rippling waters, several small birds in flight, and scalloped edging under the lip.

I told the group that the cup had been in our family for generations. I mentioned that after examining the distinctive markings on the bottom, appraisers felt confident that it originated in France during the mid-1800s and was worth upward of $10,000 dollars at auction.

I offered to pass it around, but the first person in line was reluctant to take it, fearing they might accidentally drop it. After some coaxing, they gently clutched it in both hands as if it were a baby bird, examined it closely, then nervously passed it on. Each person in turn handled it with enormous care.

I leaned over the last person, took back the cup when they had finished, then callously tossed it in the air. It arched upward, paused momentarily at the high point, then quickly descended, hitting the hard wood floor and smashing into a couple dozen jagged pieces.

Everyone gasped and stared in horror at the sprawling wreckage. A few moments of stunned silence followed. I then told them the truth. I had actually purchased the cup at the local department store the day before for about $3.00 and dropped it on purpose to make a point – *the more we value something, the better we'll take care of it.*

Many people are currently treating their bodies in very unfortunate, callous ways. As a result, obesity, diabetes, heart disease, and myriad other self-inflicted ailments are reaching epidemic proportions. Much of it can be traced to the fact that we vastly undervalue the wonders of our physical frame.

The Scriptures teach that we are "fearfully and wonderfully made" (Psalm 139:14, NKJV). God has given each of us a priceless gift of an amazingly complex body. The more we value it, the better we'll most likely take care of it.

An important key to valuing what we have been given is to understand more fully the body's intricacies and inner workings. In this lesson we'll focus on a few aspects of our biology that will hopefully establish a foundation for valuing God's gift more deeply and handling it more carefully. The following are some facts that can evoke an inner "Wow!" in all of us. Remember, these facts are not about some marvel outside of yourself like a Grand Canyon or space ship; they are all about you.

> *The more we value something, the better we'll take care of it.*

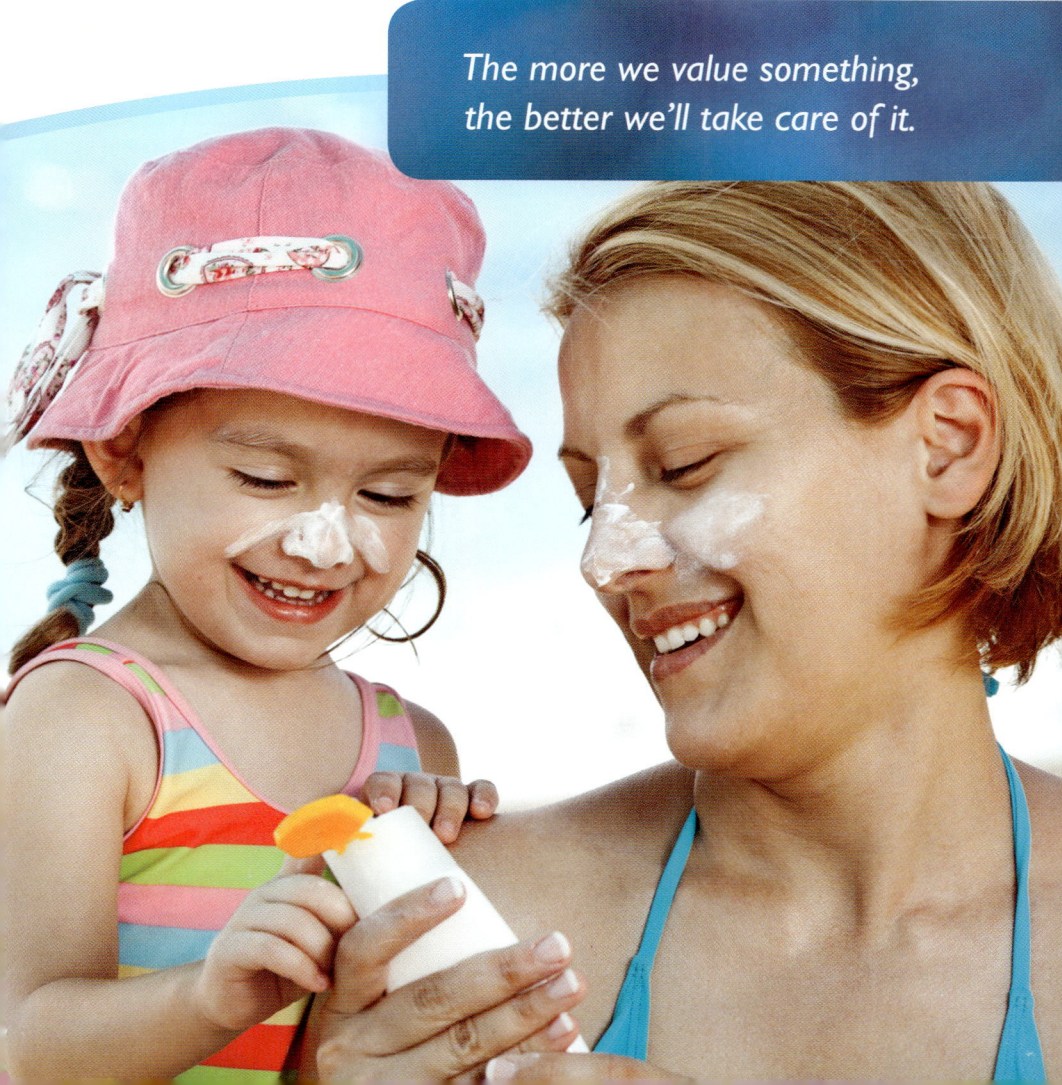

The average human body has about 75 *trillion* cells.[3] It is easy to read that number much too quickly. Let's pause and give it some thought. So how big is *one* trillion? That's a "1" followed by twelve zeros. Consider the following:

If we used seconds as a comparison, a *million* seconds is 11.5 days, a *billion* seconds is over thirty-one years, and a *trillion* seconds is over 31,000 years.[4] If you earned $40,000 per year, it would take twenty-five million years to earn one trillion dollars.[5] "One trillion pennies stacked on top of each other would make a tower about 870,000 miles high – the same distance obtained by going to the Moon, back to Earth, then to the Moon again."[6]

A trillion of anything is truly beyond imagining. And the number of cells in your very own body is about seventy-five times that number!

What other wonders lie within us? If you placed all of the blood vessels in your body end to end, they would cover about sixty thousand miles.[7] That's over two times around the Earth! Your tiny vessels would stretch all the way across the Atlantic Ocean, France, Italy, Slovenia, Croatia, Serbia, Romania, Ukraine, part of Russia, across Kazakhstan, China, South Korea, Japan, the Pacific Ocean, and the United States, over two times.

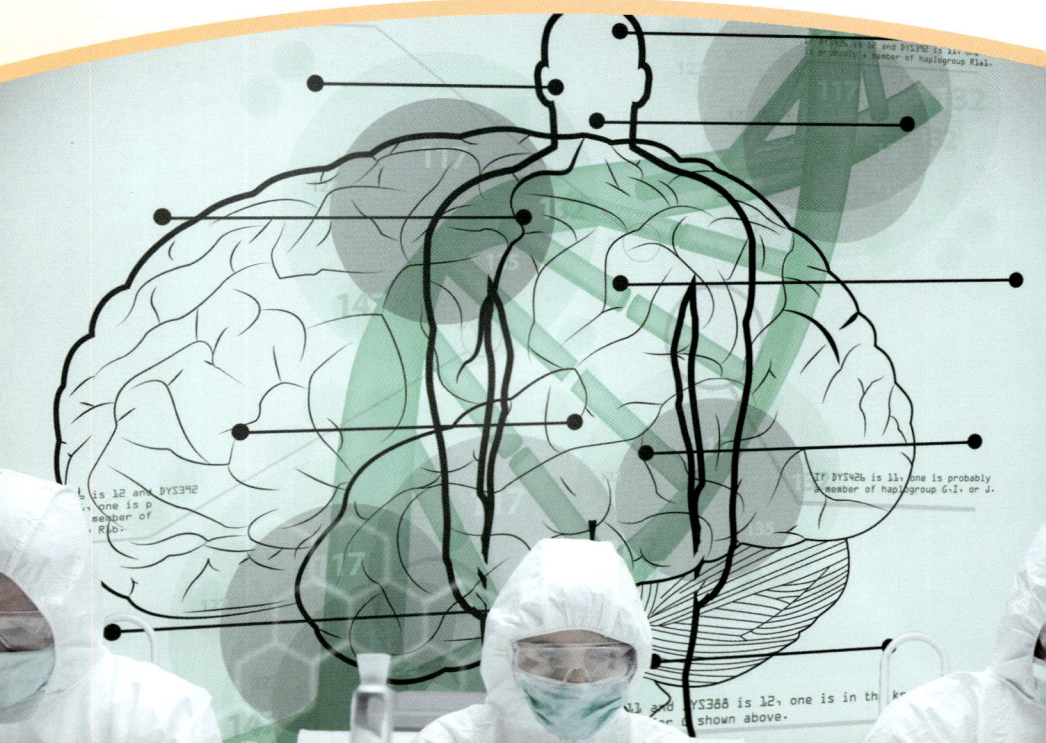

Your heart will beat without stopping about 100,000 times each day and over thirty-five million times during the next twelve months.[8] Over an average lifetime, it will pump enough blood to fill three super tankers.[9] Every extra pound you gain adds seven miles of new blood vessels that your heart has to pump blood through.[10]

Each cell in the human body contains six to eight feet of DNA (deoxyribonucleic acid), which has all the instructions for making another you.[11] If printed out, those instructions would fill one thousand one-thousand-page books.[12] Stretched out end to end, all of the DNA *from all of the cells in the body* would reach from the Earth to the Moon and back again over 100,000 times![13]

The human brain contains over one hundred billion nerve cells called neurons.[14] Each neuron can connect to thousands other neurons, resulting in a network of hundreds of trillions of linkages. Stephen Smith, PhD, professor of molecular and cellular physiology, observes, "In a human, there are more than 125 trillion synapses [connections] just in the cerebral cortex alone." That is approximately the number of stars in 1,500 Milky Way galaxies.[15]

Your lungs contain about six hundred million tiny air sacs called alveoli. Stretched out, they would cover an area the size of a tennis court.[16]

One of the most remarkable parts of our bodies is the complex digestive system that processes all of the food that we eat. It has to convert those foods into a form our cells can ultimately use.

Digestion starts in the mouth when we chew and food is mixed with saliva. Chewing performs an important function by breaking foods into smaller pieces that are easier for the digestive system to process.

When we swallow, the mushed up food slips down our esophagus and travels into the stomach. The stomach churns the food over and over, thoroughly mixing it with various gastric juices. One of those juices is hydrochloric acid, which unravels the large, twisted protein molecules.[17] The stomach also produces mucus along its walls to protect itself from being harmed.[18]

Most of the actual digestion happens in the small intestine.[19] The liver and gallbladder contribute bile to break down fats so they can be digested further. Bile acts much like detergents do when you put greasy pans in your dishwasher.[20] The pancreas and the small intestine itself contribute very specialized enzymes that take apart carbohydrates, proteins, and fats. There are a great variety of enzymes to handle the wide range of foods that people ingest, from breads and salads to entrees and cookies.[21]

Once the food is digested, it needs to be distributed throughout our body so we can benefit. That transfer is only possible because the lining of the small intestine is designed in a very unique way. It is made up of millions of tiny folds and finger-like projections call "villi." These create a huge surface area where very small blood and lymph vessels can come in contact with the nutrients and absorb them. If the surface area of the small intestine was spread out it would equal over 2,100 square feet, the floor area of an average two-story house![22]

Any unabsorbed food flows into the five- to six-foot-long large intestine. It is estimated that there are some *one hundred trillion microorganisms* living in a person's large intestine. Some of these five hundred species of bacteria are good guys that help provide further digestion; others are not. The bad bacteria can significantly increase our risk of infection and disease unless we eat a well-balanced diet with lots of fruits and vegetables that provide adequate amounts of fiber and other nutrients.[23]

The large intestine removes water, and the waste is eventually eliminated.

Our bodies are so complex that doctors and researchers have to narrow their focus and specialize in only certain segments of the human frame. Whole lifetimes are not enough to grasp the full dimensions of even those relatively limited spheres.

The most important thing we can do to keep all of the organs and biological systems in our incredible bodies healthy is to eat healthy food. *Good nutrition is key.* Our trillions of cells need the proper fuel in order to function properly. Unfortunately, eating well has been pushed down the list of many people's priorities, but we all deserve to give healthy eating the importance it requires.

Imagine that every person in the world got a new car free when they turned eighteen. No strings attached. No hidden fees. No tiny clauses in the contract. You sign, it's yours. They are provided by a very wealthy benefactor.

They are called "Life Cars." There are some variations in color, shape, and size, but beyond those exterior considerations, they are all the same inside. Same engine, transmission, steering, suspension, electrical, exhaust, fuel system, cooling system, brakes, etc. Intricate. High-tech. High-performance.

It is called a "Life Car" because it is the only one you get until you die. You cannot purchase another. It's this car or nothing for as long as you live. It needs to be fueled each day. All gas stations offer three different grades of fuel:

1. Fast Gasoline
2. Mixed Gasoline
3. Best Gasoline

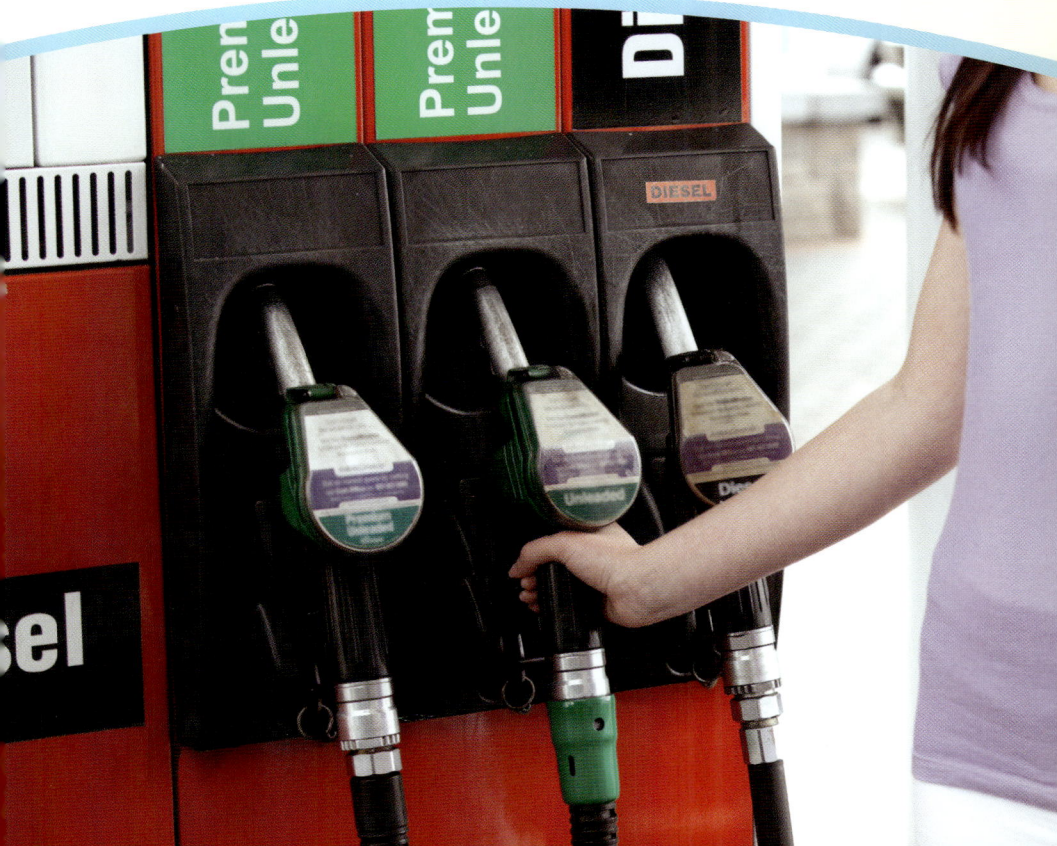

FAST GASOLINE

This is the fastest pump by far. It is very low grade, but you can fill your tank in under five minutes. It appeals to busy people who are master multitaskers. The fuel smell is intoxicating. One whiff and you've got to come back for more. As far as your car is concerned, the stuff is sludge. Periodic breakdowns are common. Over time it can cause extensive damage with big repair bills. Longtime users have to hitchhike when they get older.

MIXED GASOLINE

This pump takes longer to fill the tank – up to thirty minutes – which is definitely a challenge for people in a hurry. It is roughly a mixture of equal parts low- and high-grade fuel. It avoids several of the damaging effects of Fast Gas, but not all. It slows down performance and cuts back significantly on mileage. Other cars eventually pass you on hills. Repair bills increase over time, and car longevity is reduced.

We all get one life, and we choose the fuel.

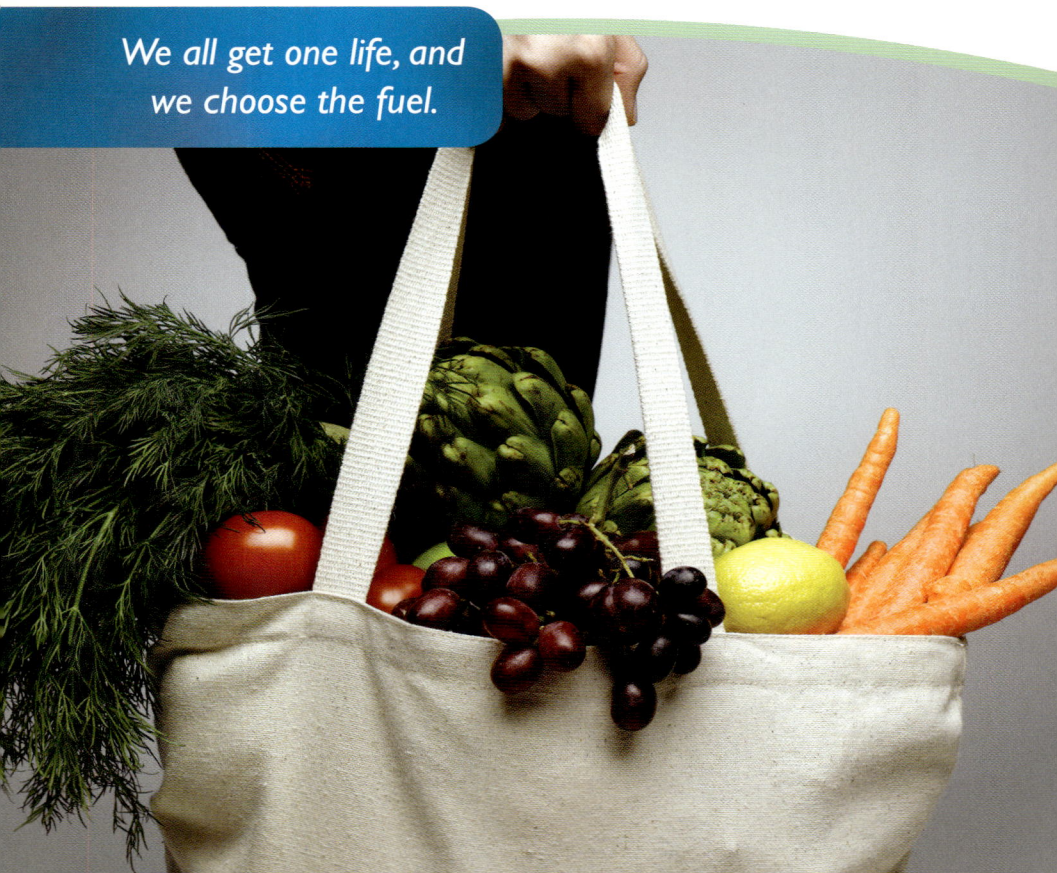

BEST GASOLINE

As the name implies, Life Cars love this fuel. The downside is that this pump is the slowest of them all, taking up to one hour to fill up. Most people who use this grade have familiarized themselves with the car's maintenance manual. They know the guidelines and the benefits. They also love the very low repair bills, great mileage, and the thrill of passing most cars on the highway. They use Mixed Gas now and then, but mostly not.

The lesson – we all get one life, and we choose the fuel. How well our bodies operate depends to a very large extent on the type of nutritional fuel we decide to utilize.

The various organs and systems in our body live under a benevolent dictatorship headed by the brain. The brain chooses what we eat, and the rest of our innards have to live with the consequences. Sometimes the brain does the smart thing. But sometimes it acts like our crazy uncle Benny and makes very debilitating selections.

The brain can make choices based on emotion and expediency. It can be easily swayed by enticing visuals and tricked by nefarious marketers. It can even get addicted to certain unhealthy foods.

The organs and biological systems can complain to each other, but they have no access to decision making. Once in a while they'll march around with signs that say, "Cerebral Cortex Unfair to Workers," but it never seems to do much good.

What we need is a more democratic decision-making process. We can make that happen. We can change from a benevolent dictatorship to a much healthier democracy by stopping for a moment before deciding what to put in our mouths and asking, "How would my internal organs vote?"

Even more importantly, we can ask ourselves, "What would honor the amazing human frame I have been given?" Honoring God's gift does not mean perfection. It means increasingly choosing good foods more often than those that are detrimental. It means choosing to continue on the journey toward the healthy, abundant life he longs for all of us to experience.

DISCUSSION

What fact about the human body in this lesson did you find most impressive? Why?
....
....

How many different brain functions can you identify in the simple act of touching the tip of your index finger to the tip of your nose?
....
....

Besides what is in this lesson, what other amazing facts do you know about the human body?
....
....

If you were to specialize in studying some aspect of biology, what would it be? Why?
....
....

How can being more aware of our body's complexity influence our food choices?
....
....

What would it take for you to use "Best Gasoline" more often?
....
....

What part of your schedule hinders you the most from taking more time to savor what you eat? How can that be adjusted?
....
....

What does your brain usually think about the most when it is deciding what to eat?
....
....

SHARING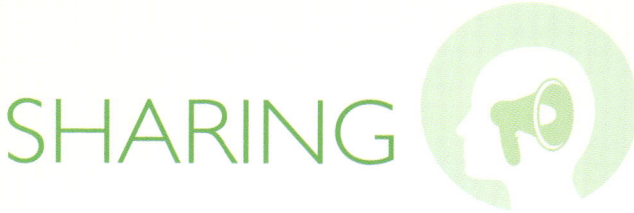

OPPORTUNITY #1

This section is about an opportunity for you to be a blessing to someone outside of your small group and to also deepen the impact of the lesson on your own life. The group is encouraged to discuss at the end of each meeting what aspects of the lesson they might like to share with someone at home, work, or in the community if the opportunity arises. *There is "An Abundant Living Thought" at the end of each lesson as one possibility of something to pass along.*

Start each day asking God to provide opportunities to share and then keep your radar up.

You can be an ambassador and reach people with the good news that abundant living is available to all.

ABUNDANT LIVING THOUGHT

God has given each of us a priceless gift of an amazingly complex body. The more we value it, the better we'll most likely take care of it.

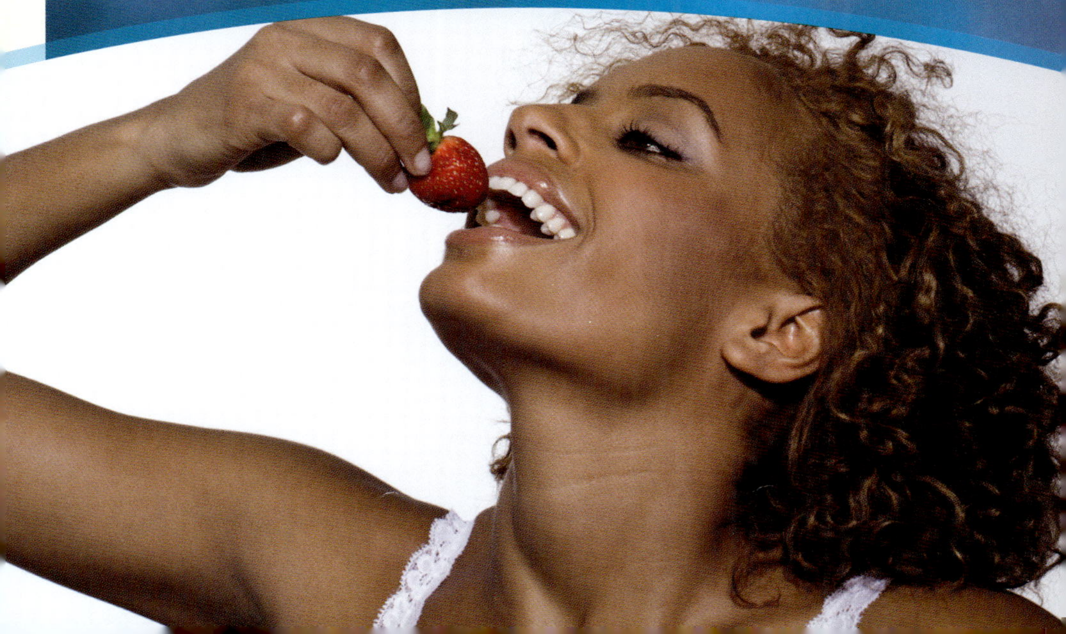

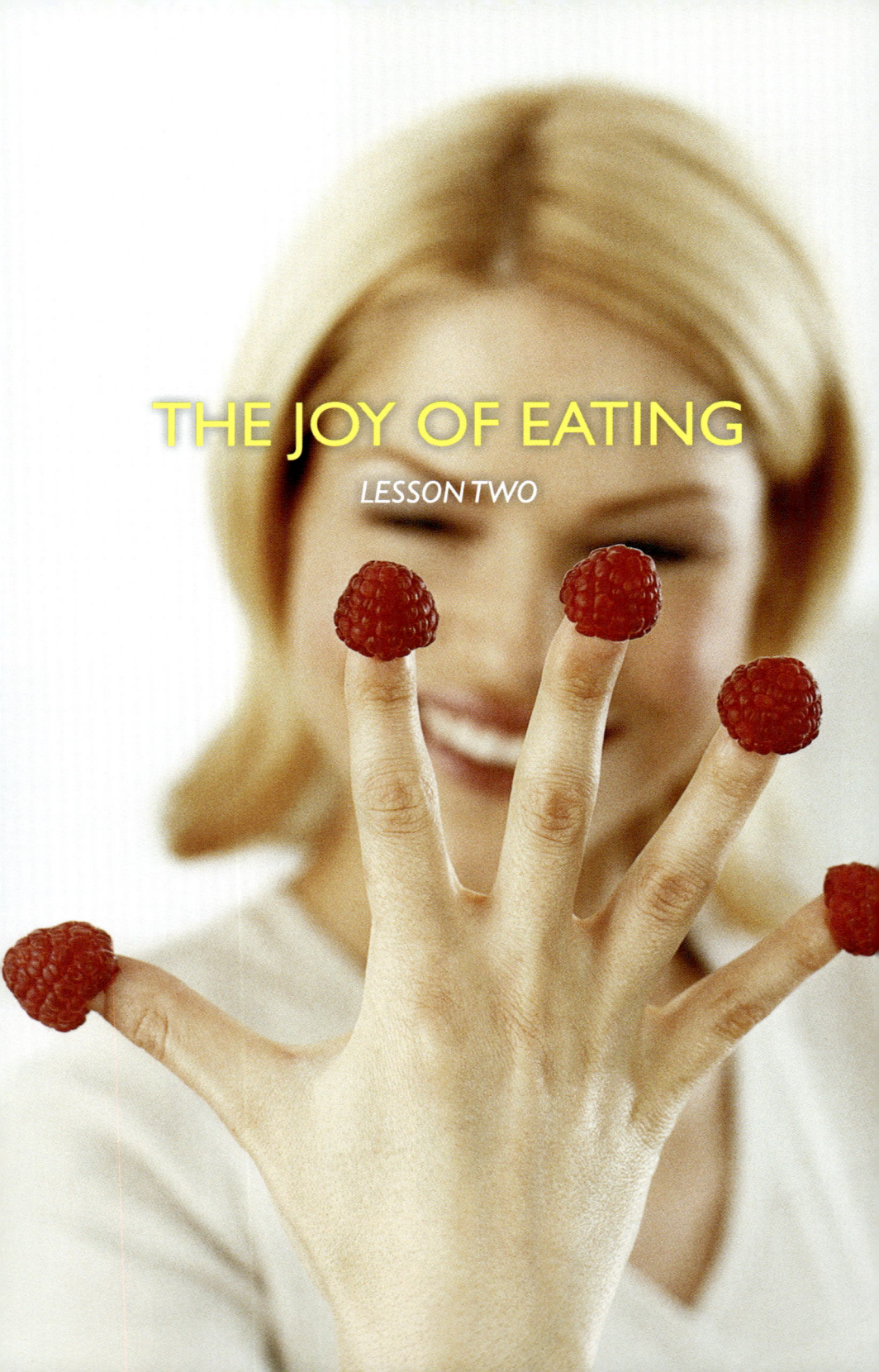

WARM UP

Feedback: In what ways did God open the door last week for you share some part of the lessons with someone else?

....
....
....
....

Choose one or both questions to discuss (if in group setting) or write out your answers on a separate sheet (for individual use):

1. **What is one of the best rewards anyone could give you?**[24]

....
....
....

2. **What book would you highly recommend to others? Why?**[25]

....
....
....

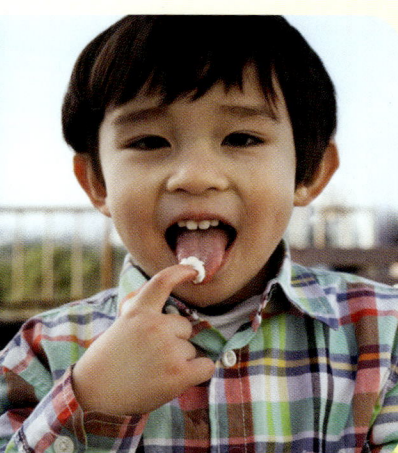

"God gave you the sense of taste to enhance your life."
DES CUMMINGS JR., PhD

DISCOVERY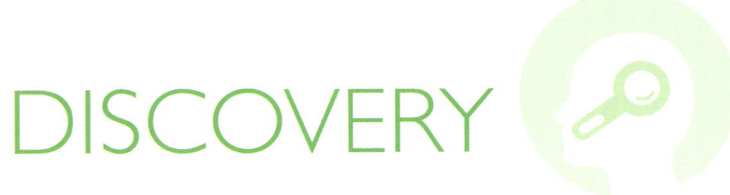

I tried to learn piano between the ages of ten and eleven. My original motivation was a love of music. My first love was saxophone, but everyone told my mother that I needed a foundation in piano first, so she found a kindly teacher and got me enrolled.

A young lady named Carol carpooled with us to the lessons. She came from China and practiced diligently, very diligently. Me . . . not so much. Learning all of the scales and fingerings was boring, and those eighty-eight keys looked terribly daunting.

Carol's lesson always came first. I'd sit on the couch listening with fear and trepidation as she breezed through the assigned pieces. Our elderly teacher gave her a big fat gold star after the first try almost every time. When my turn came to play the same piece, there were moments of flow, flashes of musicality, but mostly hit and miss. When I finished a song, she'd scribble lots of starless instructions in the margins.

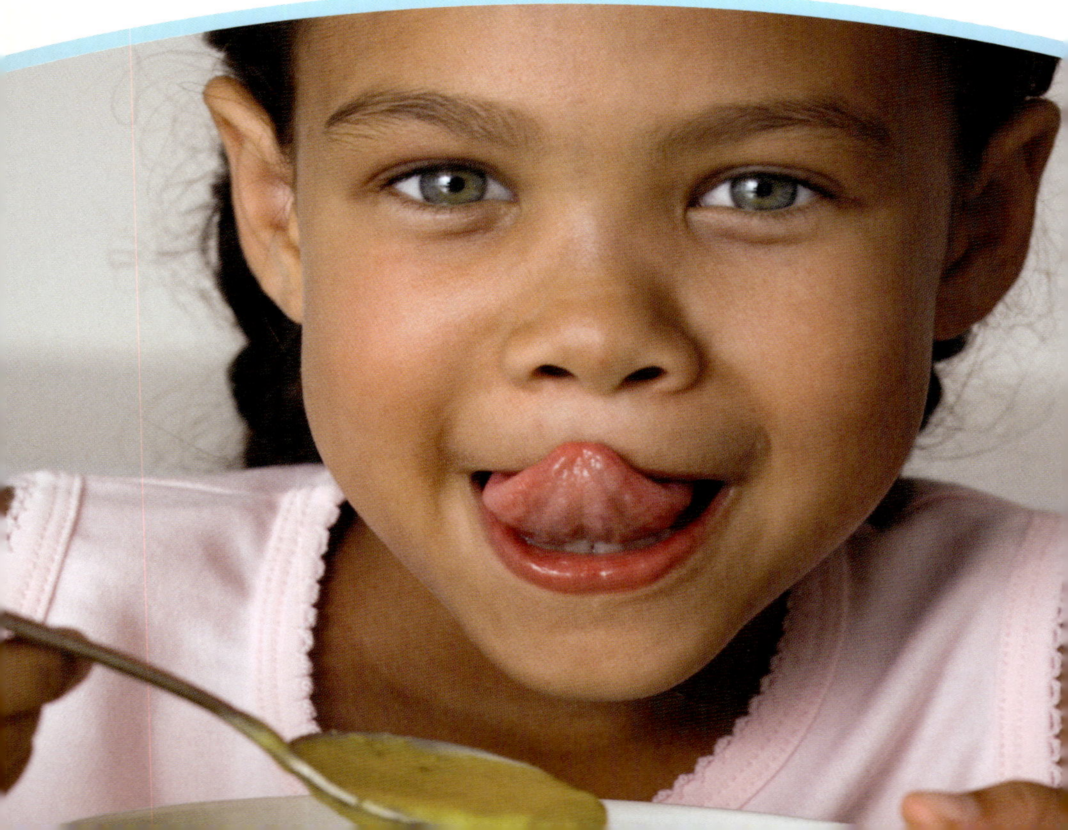

Between sessions, I'd peer at the teacher's notations and the new assignments, trying to make my fingers do what my mind envisioned, but I continued to fumble. When I sat down to play, my brain replayed lots of instructions – volume, pacing, whole notes, half notes, quarter notes, eighth notes, sixteenth notes, G clef, F clef, sharps, flats, accidentals, forte, pianissimo, codas, time signatures, hand coordination, timing, etc. *Those things are important, but along the way I lost sight of the melody.* I eventually got so caught up in the technical aspects of playing that I began to lose interest in music altogether.

That same kind of thing can happen when it comes to eating. It is certainly very important to think about fat, sugar, calories, getting the proper amounts of carbohydrates, proteins, grains, fruits, vegetables, vitamins, minerals, etc. The better we understand these issues, the better our choices are going to be.

But as we consider all the various details of good nutrition, we must not lose sight of the foundational goal of *enjoying eating.* That is the melody to which we need to be constantly attuned. According to Ellyn Satter, dietitian and therapist, "When the pleasure goes out of eating, nutrition suffers."[26] Without enjoyment, motivation can be dramatically reduced, and even the best nutritional goals can easily be derailed. The ability to make good choices over the long haul depends on there being an underlying sense of satisfaction and delight in the foods we choose to eat.

I am not talking about the hedonistic pleasure of "eat, drink, and be merry." I am not talking about the shallow, temporary high that comes from making a god out of taste. It is not a heedless attitude that focuses on today at the expense of tomorrow.

I am talking about a broader, deeper sense of enjoyment that takes pleasure in both the sensory aspects of eating and the knowledge that we are ingesting foods that will serve us well. Such considered enjoyment holds the key to making consistently good nutritional choices over time.

Foods that seem like medicine will eventually drop off our shopping list. Food selections that are driven by oughts, shoulds, and guilt trips will fade from our pantries and refrigerators. Foods with staying power must satisfy both our palette and our yearning to thrive in body, mind, and spirit.

The following are some suggestions for how to find true enjoyment in healthy eating.

1. **Know that we were designed by God to enjoy food.**
God didn't design us to graze all day like cows or eat one meal a month like a python. Our digestive system is engineered to space out our eating just enough to make it something we look forward to on a regular basis.[27]

We were created to take delight in the process of eating. Our tongues can distinguish various tastes such as sweet, sour, bitter, and salty.[28] Flavor is different than taste and comes more from our sense of smell, which can perceive hundreds of nuances. Genes, appearance, and prior experience with certain foods play a role as well.[29]

Food also brings us joy as we consider its source. Every meal can be a happy reminder of the God who provides so abundantly. Food becomes the vehicle to draw our thoughts upward to him. It points to the fact that he takes care of us in so many ways.

The Jewish nation in the Old Testament celebrated three major religious festivals that were originally tied to various harvests. There was the *Feast of Firstfruits* for the springtime barley harvest. Next came the summer *Feast of Harvest* in connection with the ripened wheat.[30] Finally there was the *Feast of Ingathering* in the autumn when olives, grapes, and other fruits were picked. This third feast was especially joyous, being the final harvest of the year. In fact, it came to be called "The Season of Joy."[31] The Israelites considered the availability of food and sustenance as a powerful reason to thank God, to rejoice in him, and so can we.

2. **Focus primarily on adding foods rather than on deleting them.**[32]
Let healthy foods crowd out unhealthy ones. If we eat more beneficial foods first, we will desire detrimental ones less. Adding makes us feel satisfied and blessed rather than deprived.

Survey your current food list. Categorize items into healthy, unhealthy, and in-between. Start by eating a little more from the healthy list. Next, expand the items on that list once a month by discovering new foods that you enjoy. Make it a "no pressure" adventure. Take your time and experiment.

Don't eat something because you're supposed to like it; eat it because you do.[33] There are plenty of nutritious items available to fill up your plate with enjoyable foods. You simply need to discover them. You can also transform some of the foods that are not your favorites into ones that are by finding the right recipe among the many that are available. We can also learn to love certain tastes over time.

My wife Ann sent me to the market awhile back with the assignment to "find a new vegetable that looks interesting." Usually I zero in on our old staples, ignoring the rest. But as I perused the produce shelves, I was surprised by the number of varieties. I grabbed some fresh kale. I'd heard of it but had never actually eaten it (as far as I knew). Ann looked up online how to cook the dark green curly leaves, and we liked them a lot. Who knew? Our healthy list grew that day by one.

3.   Give eating the importance it deserves.
Instead of thinking of eating as a time-consuming necessity, picture it as an essential oasis. Time spent ingesting food is just as important as time spent visiting with a client or accomplishing a work-related task.

4.   Slow down the eating process itself.
Sit down to eat. Turn off the phone. Refuse to multitask. Pause for a moment of appreciation before starting. Take smaller bites. Chew thoroughly. Put the fork down between mouthfuls. Take a deep breath after each swallow. Eat with your mind and not just your mouth. You cannot eat well in a hurry.[34]

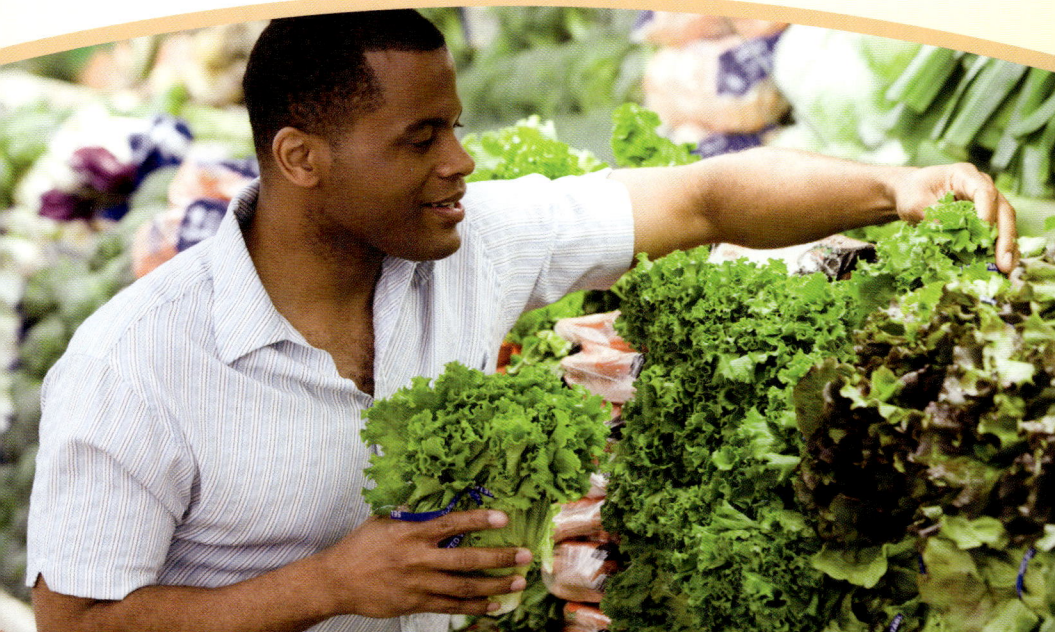

5. Periodically focus on only one piece of food.

Occasionally practice focusing on just one tiny bit of food rather than handfuls, bunches, or forkfuls. Taking delight in so little reorients the brain and opens the way for you to take much greater delight in more.[35]

For example, let's focus on just one blueberry that I select at random. It has no weight as I support it in my outstretched hand. I raise it to my nose and catch only a faint wisp of aroma.

In the mouth, I can test its firmness by exerting increasing pressure with my teeth. I can feel it bend inward like squeezing a blown-up balloon. Happy anticipation grows as I exert increasing increments of force. I don't want it to burst open too quickly.

Suddenly, I stop midbite as my mind wanders to the process of growing, picking, packing, and transport. The blueberry container said "Product of Chile," and I marvel that I can have summer fruit all year long. Who is the distant, Chilean farmer who initiated this particular aspect of the food chain?

I bite a little harder, and suddenly the blueberry bursts and my mouth is sprayed with sweetness. Bits of blue covering and the inner flesh of the fruit are strewn around my mouth like shrapnel from an exceedingly soft explosion. I keep chewing to extract every ounce of taste. I then stop all activity and let the remnants linger on my tongue. The most subtle, normally unnoticed flavors now make an appearance. Eventually the sweetness fades like the spent flavor of overly chewed gum.

My tongue presses the blueberry mush against the roof of my mouth, pushes it backward, and I consciously swallow. The demolished blueberry compliantly slips down the back of my throat and begins its journey through the twists and turns of my digestive system. I just did myself a real favor because blueberries are nutritional powerhouses.[36]

By thoroughly experiencing just one blueberry, I greatly enhance the impact and delight of the other ten sitting on my cereal when I eat them at normal speed. The same can happen with one kernel of corn, one pea, one raisin, one cashew, one thin slice of carrot, or any single tiny piece of any food carefully separated from the rest.

6. Retrain your taste buds.

Our taste buds and preferences can be warped over the years by an excess of salty, sugary, oily foods. Artificial sweeteners are a big culprit here. Many of these are hundreds of times sweeter than regular sugar. If consumed regularly, as in diet sodas, we can find healthful foods such as fruits and vegetables unappealing by comparison.[37]

We need to give ourselves time to retrain. Be patient and expect a period of transition with ups and downs. Take it in small stages without guilt or judgment. You will ultimately find healthier foods to be far more tasty than unhealthy ones as you learn to tune into a host of wonderful, often subtle, smells and flavors.

7. Eat enough but not too much.

Many Americans tend to eat too much and then feel stuffed rather than pleasantly full. They then pop pills to get rid of heartburn and stomach upset. We can educate our minds to adopt a better way.

First, ditch the little voice from childhood that says we need to clean our plate. We don't! Once we have eaten enough, any leftovers need to be put in the refrigerator or tossed. If the idea of feeding part of your dinner to the garbage disposal is too repugnant, use smaller portions to begin with.

Once we've eaten enough, leftovers need to be put in the refrigerator or tossed.

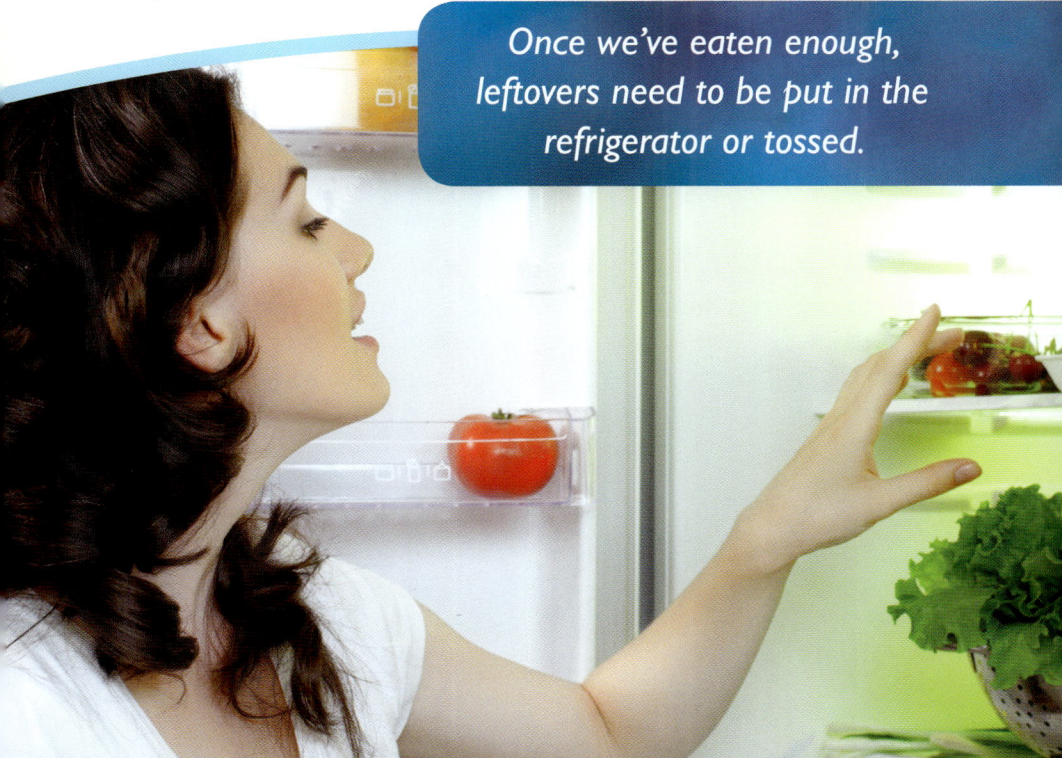

Before you eat, evaluate how hungry you are according to the following scale:

1. Very hungry, cranky, low energy, lots of stomach growling
2. Pretty hungry, stomach is growling a little
3. Satisfied, neither hungry nor full
4. A little full, pleasantly full
5. Feeling stuffed

Don't allow yourself to get to level 1 before eating. Otherwise you'll be so consumed with shoveling in food that you'll lose perspective. To keep that from happening, avoid skipping meals and get a healthy snack at midmorning and midafternoon. At meals, eat high-fiber foods first so you'll feel full longer. You'll also be less likely to fill up on lower quality items. It may be easier for some people to schedule more small meals throughout the day than the typical three.

Check in with yourself while you are eating and ask, "How full am I getting?" It can take up to twenty minutes for your stomach to bring your brain up to date on the eating process. So learn to pay more attention to what your body is telling you before you speed past the exit sign marked "Enough." Drinking some water before eating can give the signal a head start.[38] Ideally you'll be at 2 when you sit down to a meal. Stop eating when you get to 3 or 4.[39]

Kathy Nichols states, "The ironic part is that the more we truly enjoy the food, the less we eat of it. Fully experiencing the sensations allows us to be satisfied much sooner. When you are paying attention to the experience, you know when it is enough."[40]

The apostle John wrote, "I pray that you may enjoy good health and that all may go well with you, even as your soul is getting along well" (3 John 1:2, NIV). Such enjoyment of health can come as we experience the joy of eating the nutritious foods God has so abundantly provided.

NOTES:

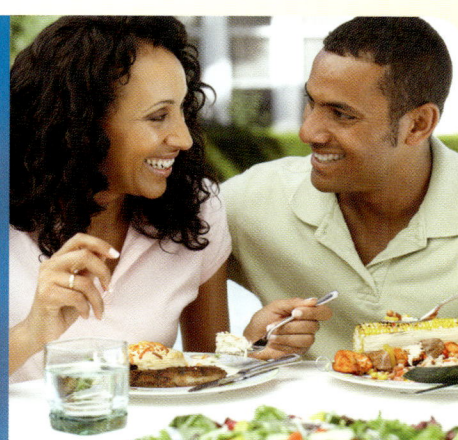

Eat with your mind and not just your mouth. You cannot eat well in a hurry.

DISCUSSION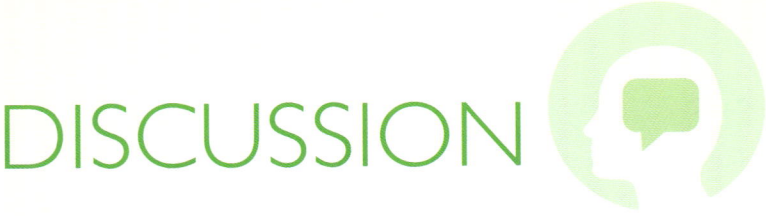

Describe one of the best meals you've ever had. Why did you enjoy it so much?

What meal do you most enjoy cooking for guests? Describe.

Why do you think focusing primarily on what foods to delete doesn't work well over time?

Is eating more of an oasis or a time-consuming necessity for you? Why?

What does it mean to you to "savor" your food? How can you do that more?

Do you currently eat any healthy foods that you do not enjoy? Are there alternatives that you do like?

What was your reaction to the description in the lesson of slowly eating one blueberry?

What signals can you listen to that would help you to not become "stuffed" when you eat?

SHARING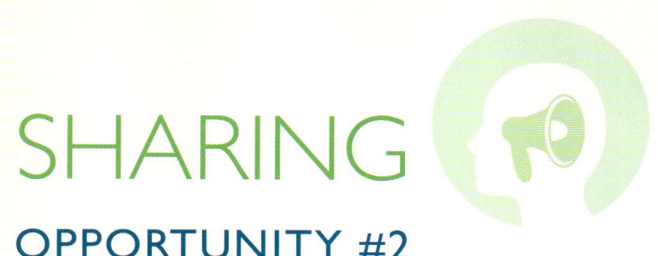

OPPORTUNITY #2

- Pray for God to open the way for you to share something from these lessons to help someone else.
- Keep your radar up each day for opportunities.

ABUNDANT LIVING THOUGHT

Don't eat something because you're supposed to like it; eat it because you do.

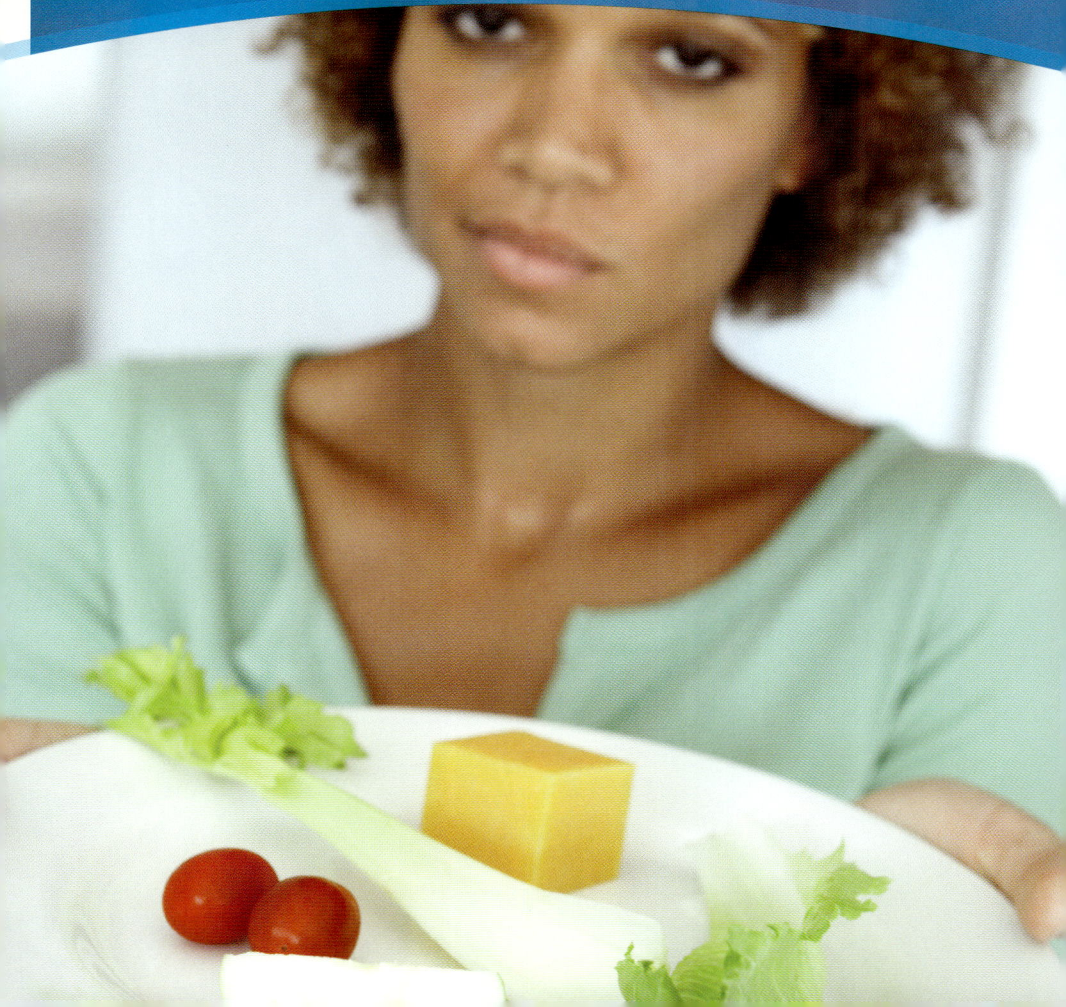

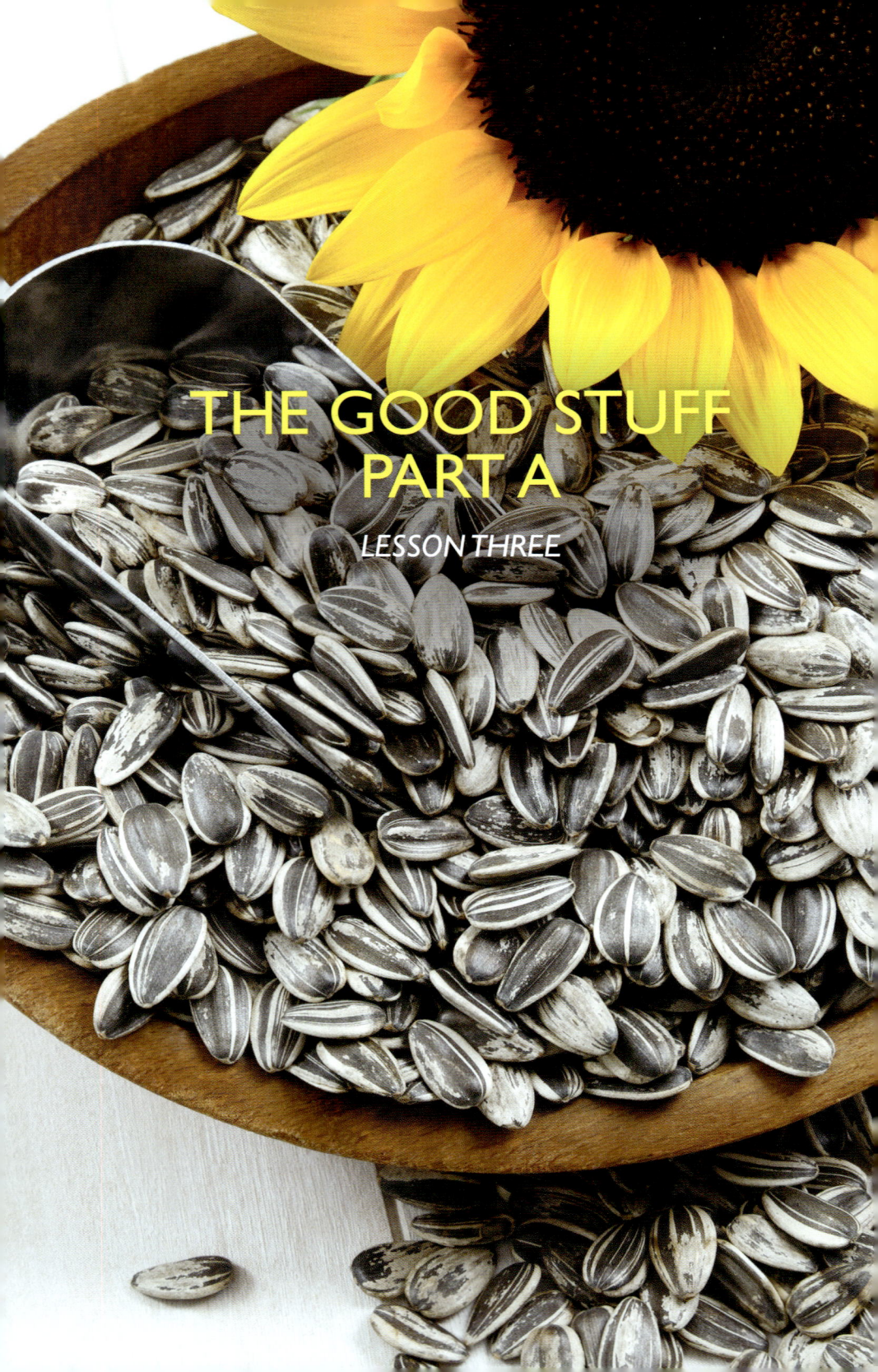

THE GOOD STUFF PART A

LESSON THREE

WARM UP

Feedback: In what ways did God open the door last week for you share some part of the lessons with someone else?

....
....
....
....

Choose one or both questions to discuss (if in group setting) or write out your answers on a separate sheet (for individual use):

1. **If you chose to write a book, what would the subject be?**[41]

....
....
....

2. **If you were invited to a costume party, what would you come as and why?**[42]

....
....
....

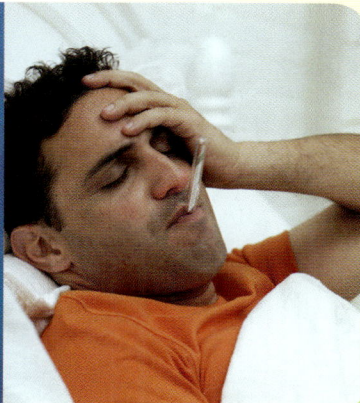

"Those who think they have no time for healthy eating will sooner or later have to find time for illness."

EDWARD STANLEY

DISCOVERY

A few miles south of Naples, Italy, lies the quaint coastal town of Pioppi. It is located picturesquely in the middle of the Cilento National Park. It boasts award-winning beaches, palm-lined promenades overlooking the sea, old traditional mansions, a scenic piazza, and cozy cafés. It is one of many little gems along the famous Amalfi coast.[43]

Perhaps Pioppi's greatest claim to fame is being the home of the well-known "Mediterranean Diet." When a researcher from America visited the town in the 1940s and '50s, he discovered that the citizens there enjoyed an exceptionally high level of health and vitality that stood in stark contrast to so much of the Western world. After lengthy study, he concluded that their diet played a major role. It consisted mostly of vegetables, fruits, whole grains, beans, berries, olives, and olive oil. World-wide attention was eventually drawn to what was not so much a "diet" as a way of life not only for the citizens of Pioppi, but for much of the rest of Italy as well.[44]

> *For a healthy eating strategy to be successful, it has to be simple, practical, flexible, and sustainable.*

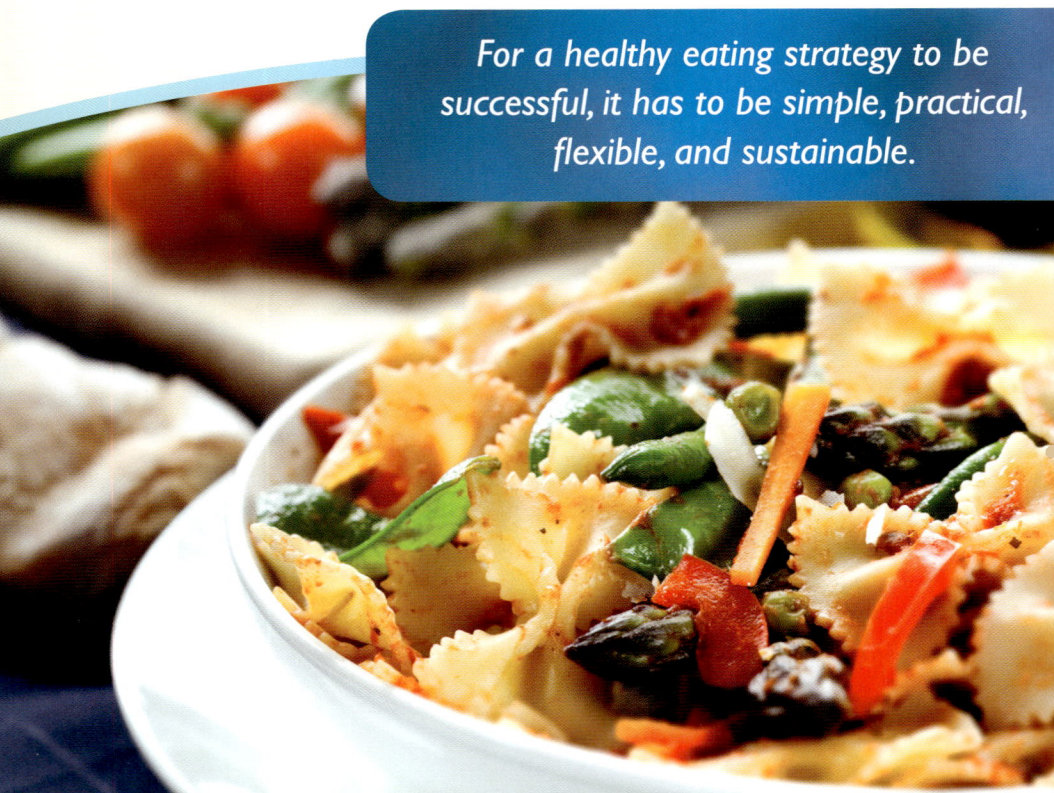

Since that time, however, there has been a dramatic change. Members of the younger generation in the town of Pioppi and elsewhere in Italy are making very different dietary choices than those of their grandparents and great-grandparents. They are taking an unhealthy turn toward highly refined and processed foods.[45]

Dr. Angelo Pietrobelli, associate professor of pediatrics and nutrition at the University of Verona, observes "Unfortunately, in particular among adolescents, they try to avoid [the] Mediterranean diet because they try to 'imitate' the US diet." He states that, sadly, up to 36 percent of twelve- to sixteen-year-olds are now either overweight or obese.[46] The problem is quickly spreading to other countries such as Greece and Spain.[47]

The low-quality food these young people are now so vigorously consuming has been prevalent throughout the United States for decades. These "fast foods" and highly processed products laden with sugar and saturated fat are major contributors to America's deepening health problems. The picture is rather grim. According to the Centers for Disease Control, 70 percent of all deaths in the United States are from chronic diseases. One person is killed by heart disease every minute. Cancer takes another 1,500 lives each day. These two diseases combined claim over one million lives annually.

Two out of three adults are either overweight or obese. Obesity among children and adolescents has almost tripled since 1980.[48] In the last ten years, the incidence of diabetes has increased by a whopping 90 percent. It now affects 25.8 million people, about 8.3 percent of the population. In addition, it is estimated that 79 million Americans, twenty years of age or older, have prediabetes.[49]

How terribly sad, especially when we realize that these and other chronic diseases can be largely prevented through simply changing our eating habits. It could, in fact, be said that the leading cause of death in the United States is poor nutritional choices.[50]

Eating healthy foods is the most powerful weapon available to combat illness. What people put on their plate can have a far greater positive effect on our population's overall health than popping pills or going under the surgeon's knife. The future can be very different through heightened awareness, increased knowledge, and an ongoing commitment to good nutrition.

According to the American Diabetes Association, "Eating well to maintain a healthy weight is one of the most important things you can do to lower your risk for type 2 diabetes and heart disease."[51]

The American Heart Association adds, "Eating the right foods is important, especially when you have heart disease. A heart-healthy diet and physical activity help you maintain good health and reduce your risk of future heart problems."[52]

The American Institute for Cancer Research offers the following hopeful comment, "You can start lowering your cancer risk at your very next meal. Experts recommend that our diets revolve around plant foods, such as vegetables, fruits, whole grains, and beans."[53]

What often keeps people from adopting better eating habits is their perception that it's way too complicated. They can think of the myriad diets and complex eating plans that require them to do a lot of calculating and counting and weighing and measuring, and they feel overwhelmed.

It can be too much of a hassle to constantly have to worry about consulting charts and honing in on precise target amounts. People may have the desire, but the hectic pace of life can make complex plans unworkable.

For a healthy eating strategy to be successful, it has to be simple, practical, flexible, and sustainable. What we need is a lifestyle, not another twelve-week, quick-fix strategy because that doesn't usually work over the long haul.

One of the best pathways for mealtime success is very simple, yet surprisingly powerful. *All we need to do is focus on foods that have lots of fiber.*

Everyday, common, fiber-rich foods hold the key to the wellness that so many people desire. You won't find them promoted by the marketers on TV, the fast food restaurant chains, or corner convenience stores. But you can follow the beat of a different drummer, do yourself a huge favor, and choose the better way.

It turns out that if we place our primary focus on getting enough fiber in whole foods, all the other things we need begin to fall into place. If you need to lose weight, focusing on fiber-rich foods can get you there. If your weight is not an issue but you want to take your eating habits to the next level, they can provide that, too.[54]

Fiber expert Joanne Slavin, PhD, RD, a professor at the University of Minnesota in St. Paul and member of the 2010 Dietary Guidelines Advisory Committee, says, "There is no downside to eating a diet rich in fiber. And the potential health gains are significant."[55]

What makes fiber so appealing as the centerpiece of great eating is that it is found in so many wonderful, easily accessible sources. Fiber comes only from plants – primarily fruits, vegetables, beans, and whole grains – which lines up perfectly with the key elements of the old Mediterranean way of eating. *When you seek out the fiber in these four kinds of foods, you also get all the other great nutrients those foods contain.*

> *All we need to do is focus on foods that have lots of fiber.*

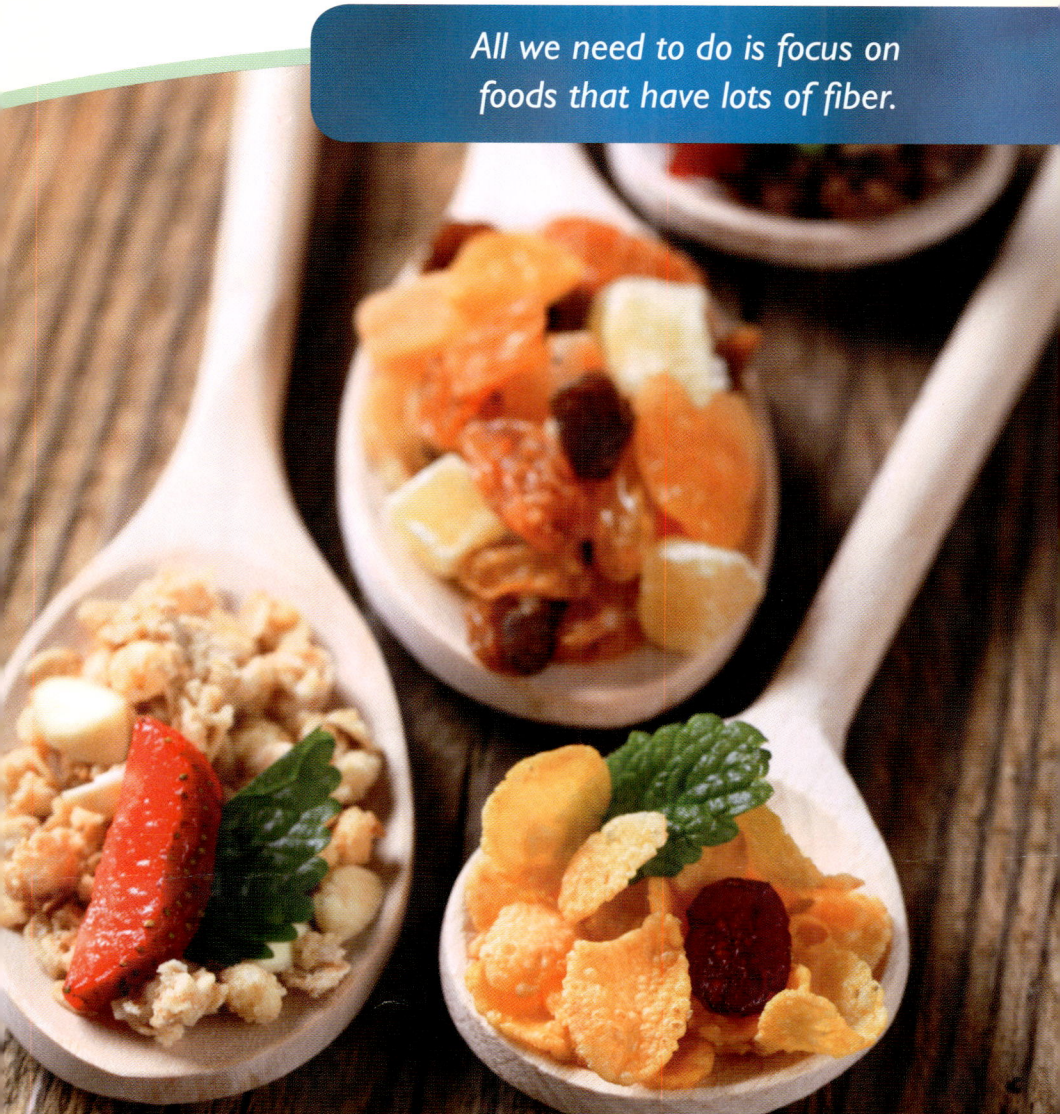

Suppose you chose to study overseas for a year in four different countries – Greece, India, China, and Kenya. You may spend lots of time hitting the books, but there is no way you're not going to be dramatically enriched by each country's culture. Your senses will absorb the experiences outside of school, and you will be irrevocably changed for the better. Even though your primary focus is a great education, everything else comes along for the ride.

Or suppose a bee was instructed to get nectar from four different kinds of flowers. Even though nectar is the main mission, it's going to come back loaded with pollen, too. It is the same way with fiber. That may be your principle focus, but when you get it from the four food types, lots of other good stuff happens to you as well. It is a package deal. One cannot be separated from the other.

Even though fiber itself essentially provides no calories and is not digested by the body, it performs numerous important roles and has a profound positive effect on our health. It helps lower cholesterol, control blood sugar levels by slowing the absorption of sugar, regulate digestion and elimination, protect against certain cancers, reduce the risk of diabetes, lower blood pressure, and reduce the threat of heart disease, to name a few.[56]

> *Success is not defined by how far you are from the ideal but by how far you have come from where you were.*

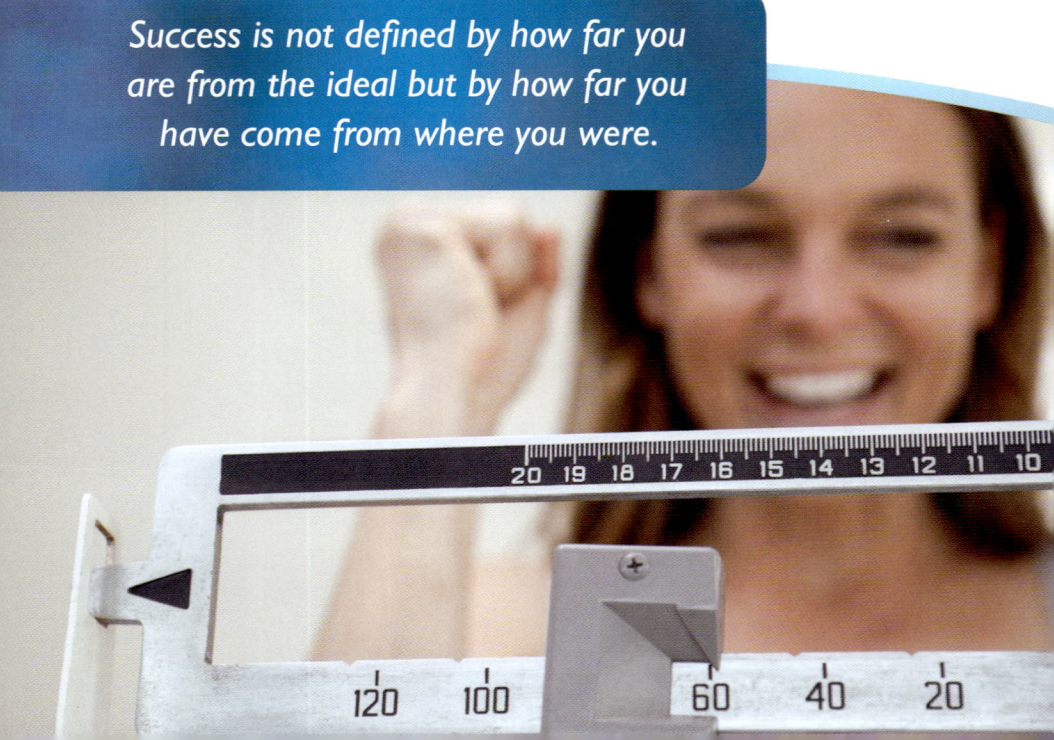

Fiber alone does not provide all the variety of health benefits we need, but fiber and the foods it comes in do. Centering on fiber simply provides a convenient, easy-to-follow way of making sure we're getting all of the great food our bodies require. There's much less hassle, a lot fewer frustrations, and minimal headaches. *When deciding what to eat, simply give priority to foods that are good sources of fiber.*

To get maximum benefit, it is essential that we make food choices *from all of the four fiber-rich sources on a daily basis – fruits, vegetables, beans, and whole grains.* All four may not show up on your plate for every meal, but at the end of the day they all need to have been eaten. You choose the combinations and the amounts that suit you best. That leaves room for literally thousands of possibilities.[57]

It is also important to eat a small handful of fiber-rich nuts and seeds each day. They do not appear on your food plate, but they need to be eaten consistently in order to gain all of the special benefits they provide. My wife and I keep a bag of nuts on the counter as a reminder to grab a handful on a regular basis.

Experts such as Andrew Weil, MD, director of the Arizona Center for Integrative Medicine at the University of Arizona, and Jeff Greenberg, MD, Chief of Cardiology and Cardiovascular Surgery at Arrowhead Hospital, recommend that in order to receive maximum benefit, the ideal is to take in thirty-five to forty grams of fiber from the foods we eat each day.[58] That is not a hard and fast rule for every person and circumstance, but it is an important target to strive toward for most people. Children would need less.[59]

Forty grams per day is far more than the eleven to fifteen grams that Americans currently get on average.[60] The closer to the ideal we come, the more benefits we receive, but every gram over fifteen each day should be cause for celebration! This is a guilt-free zone. *Success is not defined by how far you are from the ideal but by how far you have come from where you were.*

Introduce more fiber-rich foods into your eating strategy slowly or else your gastric system might get extra rumbly and bloated. Set goals for yourself such as three to five more grams every week or two. Also drink extra amounts of water because fiber absorbs water like crazy.

The highest recommendation for eating fiber-rich foods comes from God himself in the story of Creation in the Old Testament book of Genesis. He told Adam and Eve, "I give you every seed-bearing plant on the face of the whole earth and every tree that has fruit with seed in it. They will be yours for food" (Genesis 1:29, NIV). Monica Reed, MD, comments, "A vast variety of fruits, vegetables, nuts, seeds, grains, herbs, and flavorful seasonings were theirs to enjoy."[61] The first chapter of Genesis concludes, "And God saw everything that he had made, and, behold, it was very good" (Genesis 1:31, KJV). The God who made us certainly ought to know what fuel we run on best.

> *The highest recommendation for eating fiber-rich foods comes from God himself.*

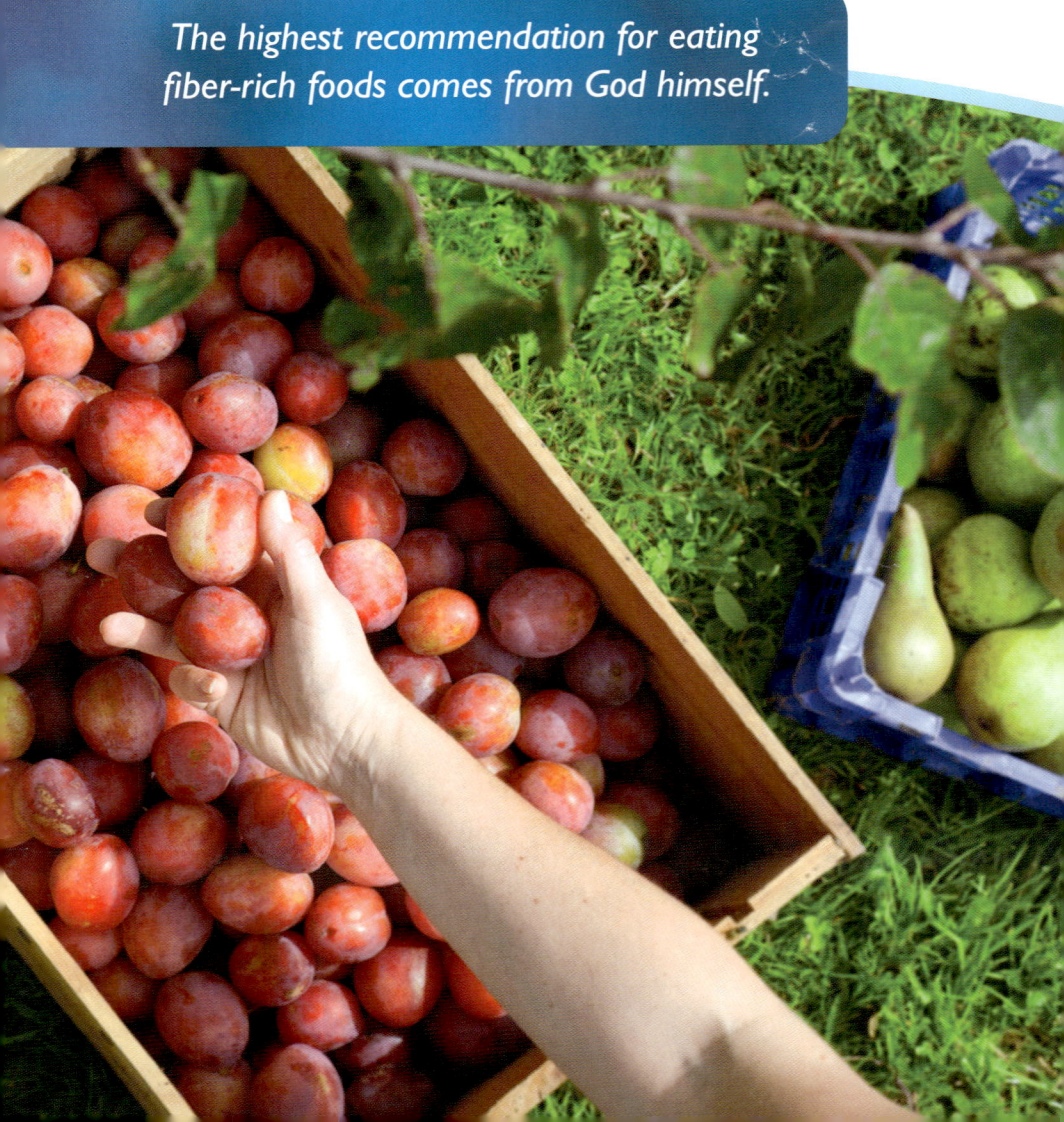

Here are some fiber numbers to get you started. The list has the name, the amount of food, and the grams of fiber.[62] Note that there is no fiber in meat, dairy, or eggs. Beans are certainly the big winner. Choose one new item from this list to add to your shopping list this week.

FRUITS
Blackberries, 1 cup, 8g
Raspberries, 1 cup, 8g
Boysenberries, 1 cup, 7g
Pear, 1 medium, 6g
Apple, 1 medium, 4g
Orange 1 medium, 4g
Banana, 1 medium, 3g
Blueberries, 1 cup, 3g
Strawberries, 1 cup, 3g
Peaches, 1 cup, 3g

VEGETABLES
Avocado, 1 medium, 13g[63]
Acorn squash, cooked, 1 cup, 9g
Broccoli, cooked, 1 cup, 5g
Sweet potatoes, cooked, 1 medium, 5g
Cauliflower, cooked, 1 cup, 5g
Carrots, cooked, 1 cup, 5g
Corn, cooked, 1 cup, 4g
Spinach, cooked, 1 cup, 4g
Beet greens, cooked, 1 cup, 4g
Swiss chard, cooked, 1 cup, 4g
Green beans, cooked, 1 cup, 4g

BEANS
Navy beans, cooked, 1 cup, 19g
Split peas, cooked, 1cup, 16g
Lentils, cooked, 1 cup, 16g
Pinto beans, cooked, 1 cup, 15g
Black beans, cooked, 1 cup, 15g
Lima beans, cooked, 1 cup, 13g
Kidney beans, cooked, 1 cup, 13g
Garbanzo beans, cooked, 1 cup, 12g
Baked beans, vegetarian, cooked, 1 cup, 10g

GRAINS
Whole grain wheat flour, 1 cup, 14g
Bulgar wheat, cooked, 1 cup, 8g
Whole wheat spaghetti, cooked, 1 cup, 6g
Barley, cooked, 1 cup, 6g
Quinoa, cooked, 1 cup, 5g
Buckwheat, cooked, 1 cup, 5g
Oatmeal, instant, cooked, 1 cup, 4g
Brown rice, cooked, 1 cup, 4g

NUTS & SEEDS[64]
Sunflower seeds, ¼ cup, 4g
Almonds, 1 ounce, 3g
Pistachio nuts, 1 ounce, 3g
Flaxseeds, 1 tbsp, 3g
Pecans, 1 ounce, 2g
Sesame seeds, 1 tbsp, ½ g

For more information about fiber in foods, visit:
http://www.mayoclinic.com/health/fiber/NU00033.
See also: http://www.puristat.com/fiber/fiberchart2.aspx.

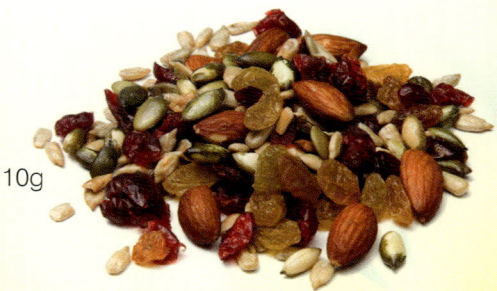

DISCUSSION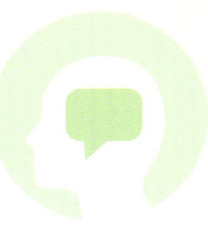

Why do you think so many people in Pioppi turned away from the Mediterranean diet?
....
....

How do you react to the fast food slogan, "Let taste be your guide?"
....
....

If you were creating a salad from four fruits, how would you make it?
....
....

Describe your favorite recipe using vegetables.
....
....

How many ways can the group think of to use beans?
....
....

How could you add five more grams of fiber to your daily diet in the next week?
....
....

How can people be more conscious of how much fiber they are getting without getting bogged down in a lot of counting?
....
....

What are some ways to get children to eat more fruits and vegetables?
....
....

SHARING

OPPORTUNITY #3:

- Pray for God to open the way for you to share something from these lessons to help someone else this week.
- Keep your radar up each day for opportunities.

ABUNDANT LIVING THOUGHT

Eating healthy foods is the most powerful weapon available to combat illness.

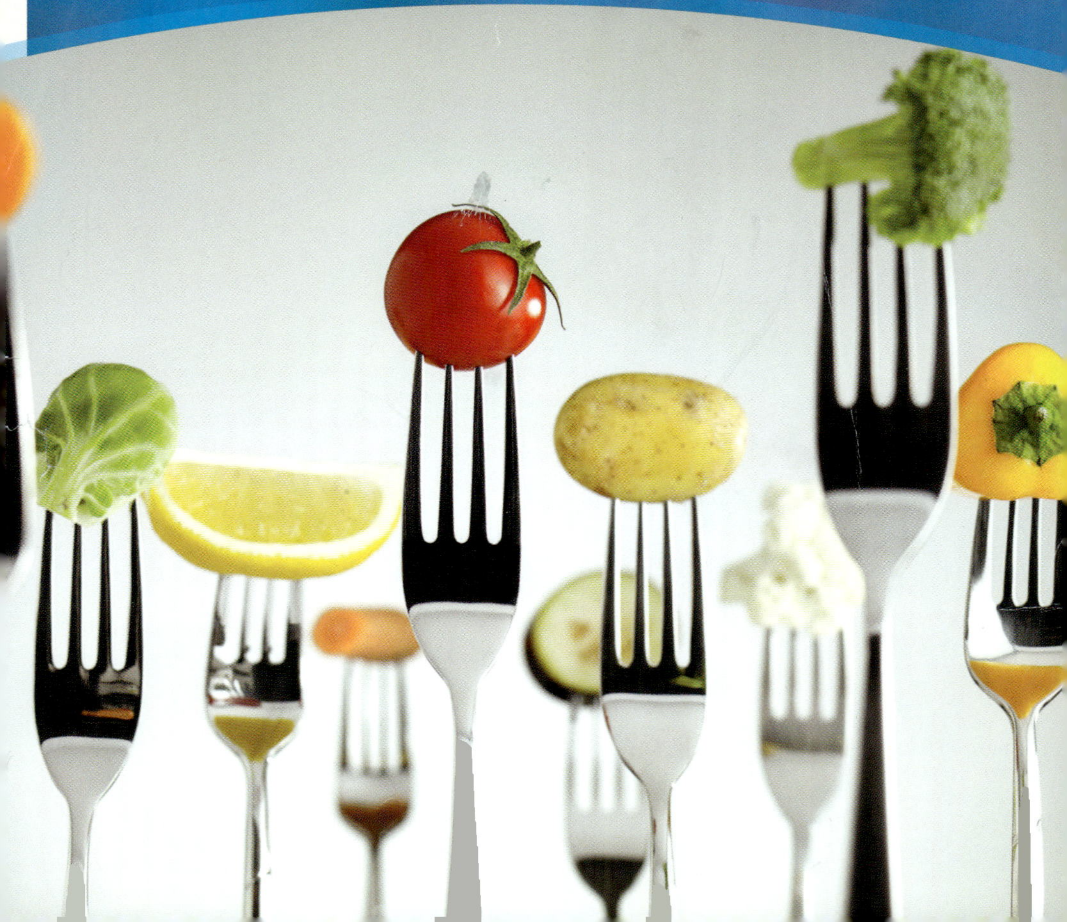

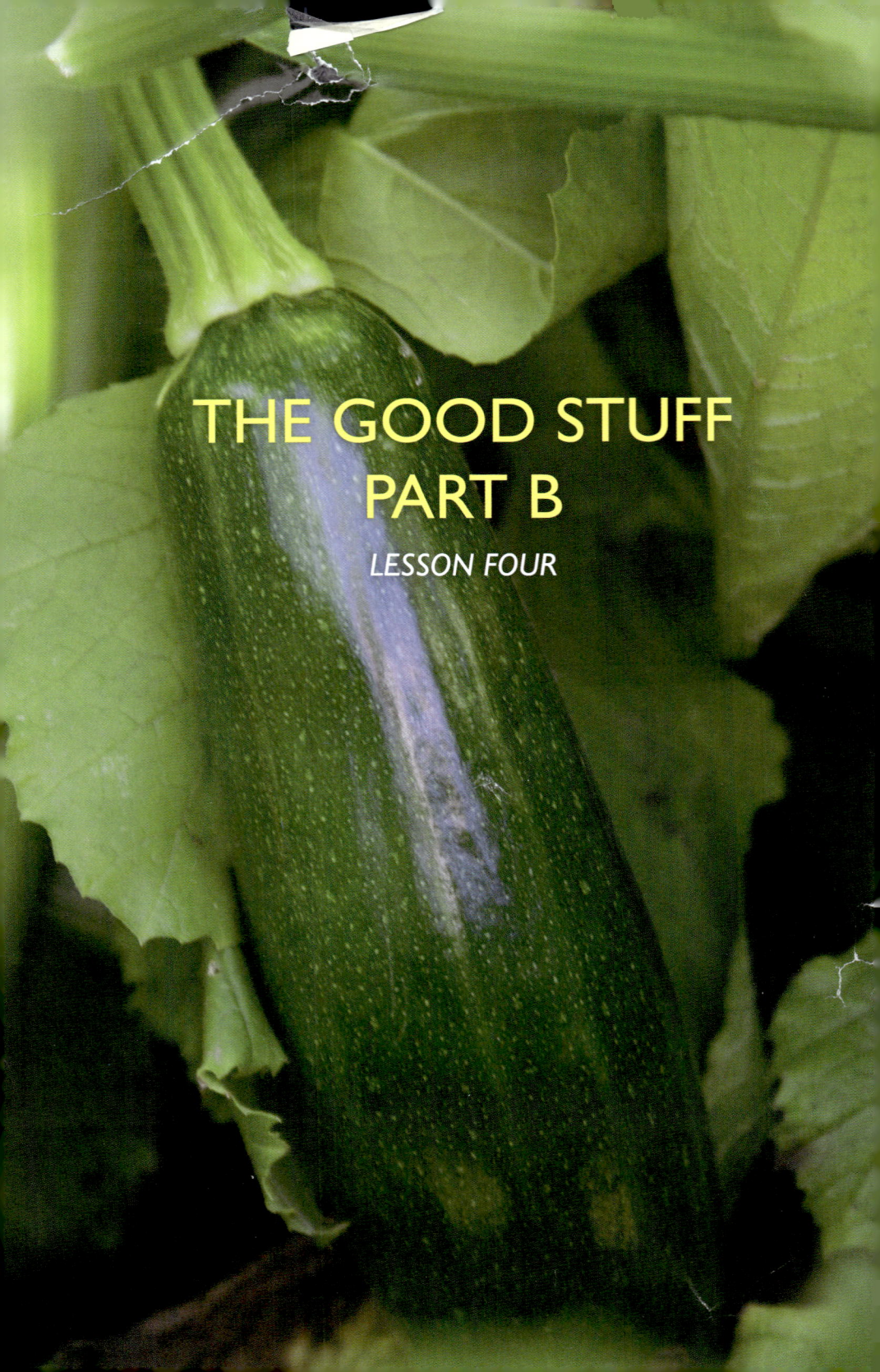

THE GOOD STUFF PART B

LESSON FOUR

WARM UP

Feedback: In what ways did God open the door last week for you share some part of the lessons with someone else?

....
....
....
....

Choose one or both questions to discuss (if in group setting) or write out your answers on a separate sheet (for individual use):

1. **What would you do tomorrow if fear was not an issue?**[65]

....
....
....

2. **What is one of the best ways you have found to relieve stress?**[66]

....
....
....

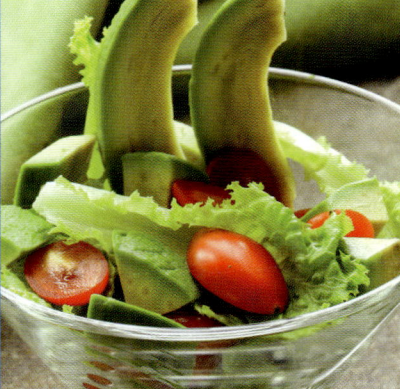

"To eat is a necessity, but to eat intelligently is an art."
LA ROCHEFOUCAULD

DISCOVERY

I have a soft spot in my heart for zucchini squash because of what happened during graduate school. My wife Ann and I had been living in our little off-campus apartment for about six months when we ran out of money for food.

Ann had a bachelor's degree in social studies but couldn't find a job. She applied everywhere, but you had to have either a master's degree or experience, and she had neither. I worked part time for the university janitorial services, cleaning anything on campus that got dirty, but that paycheck wouldn't arrive for a week and a half.

> *It wasn't difficult to eat my daily nutritional requirement of veggies when zucchini was the only food we had, but after that time of shortage I ate too many highly refined and processed foods instead.*

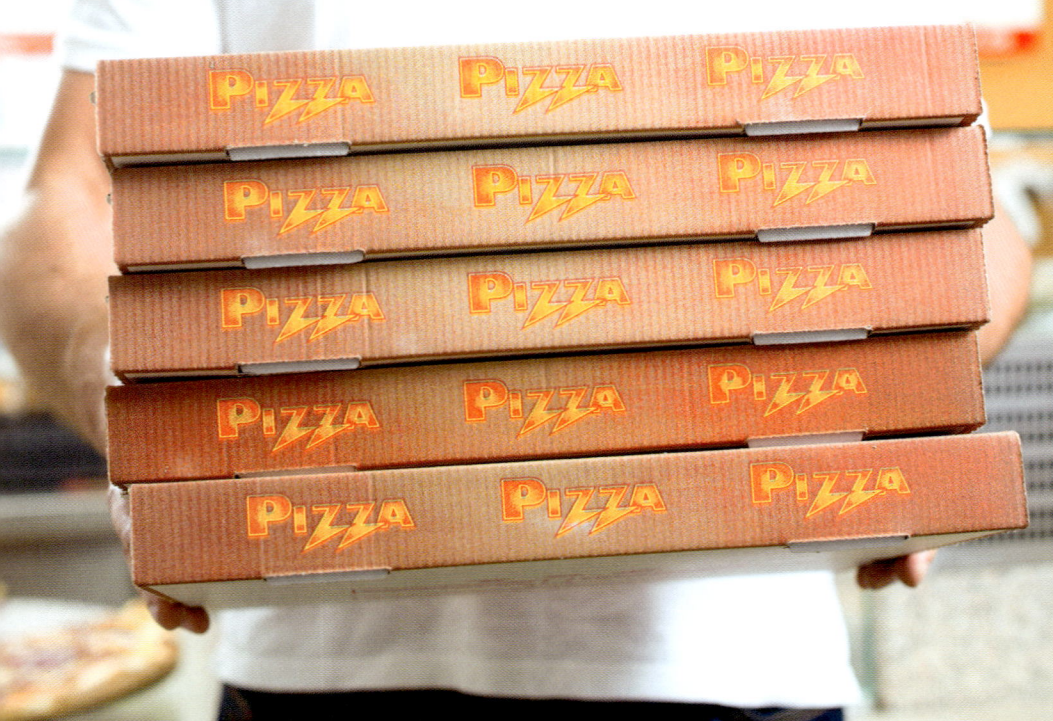

We had already drained our tiny savings, so that was a dry hole. We checked under the sofa cushions for dimes and nickels but found only a few pieces of old pizza crust. A search of the rest of the apartment for stray change turned up six pennies.

Without resources to do any shopping, we soon began rationing what little remained in the cupboards and the refrigerator. Anxiety increased as our food supply quickly shrank then ran out completely. The rumble in our stomachs grew louder. I knew of no food banks at the time that we could go to for help.

We didn't tell anyone about our plight, but we did offer a desperate prayer for some kind of assistance. The next morning, Ann went out to the mailbox in our front yard and couldn't believe her eyes. Someone had put a gigantic zucchini squash in there that stuck out about two feet. The thing was huge! She came running back, smiling and holding the immense gift overhead like a trophy.

For the next two days we ate lots of raw zucchini, fried zucchini, and baked zucchini. On the third day a letter arrived from her parents with a check for $100. The note said they had felt impressed to start sending assistance each month. It is not often that the prayers my wife and I offer are answered so dramatically, but we will be forever grateful for that one.

It wasn't difficult to eat my daily nutritional requirement of veggies when zucchini squash was the only food we had. After that time of shortage, however, the story got more checkered. Too often vegetables slipped down my priority list. To some degree, the same could have been said regarding the remaining members of the fabulous foursome – fresh fruits, whole grains, and beans. I ate too many highly refined and processed foods instead. Since learning more about the importance of fiber-rich foods and their many benefits, the trend has definitely changed for the better.

If we are going to get our full complement of these nutritious foods, they need to slowly make their way up our shopping list and become a healthful staple. Getting there can be a challenge. In this lesson we will explore some practical ways to make these foods a more prominent part of our meals. We'll look at making both (1) Wise Choices and (2) Tiny Choices.

WISE CHOICES

As you make your eating choices, it is valuable to know that fiber-rich foods contain varying amounts of calories. Within the fiber food family we can, in fact, divide them into higher-calorie and lower-calorie categories. The primary difference between the two groups is the amount of water they contain. Water has no calories, so the more water, the fewer the number of calories on board. Water takes up some of the space that calories would otherwise occupy.[67]

The most watery fiber sources are good ol' fruits and vegetables. The following chart illustrates the surprising amount of water they contain.[68]

ITEM	% WATER
FRUITS	
APPLE	84%
APRICOT	86%
BLUEBERRIES	85%
CANTALOUPE	90%
CHERRIES	81%
CRANBERRIES	87%
ORANGE	87%
PEACH	88%
STRAWBERRIES	92%

ITEM	% WATER
VEGETABLES	
BROCCOLI	91%
CABBAGE (GREEN)	93%
CAULIFLOWER	92%
CELERY	95%
CUCUMBER	96%
EGGPLANT	92%
LETTUCE (ICEBERG)	96%
PEAS (GREEN)	79%
PEPPERS (SWEET)	92%

Grapefruit is about 91 percent water, and half of one has only thirty-nine calories. Raw carrots are about 87 percent water, and half a cup has just twenty-five calories.[69]

Because you get lots of fiber with much fewer calories, fruits and vegetables are the true superstars of the nutrition world. When you can get high fiber and low calories, it just doesn't get any better than that! You can eat these foods to your heart's content without worrying about any downside.[70] They should be given the highest priority on your shopping list.

Superstar foods like these are a great help when it comes to dealing with weight. When we burn more calories than we eat, we lose weight, and superstar foods make that easier to happen. We can eat lots of them, feel full, and still use more calories than we take in.

If weight is not an issue, superstar foods make it much easier to maintain the proper poundage while treating your body to all the vitality it needs to function well. The authors of the book, *SuperSized Kids*, observe, "Surveys have found that Americans who eat the most fruits and vegetables are the least likely to be overweight."[71]

There is another group of high-fiber foods that come with higher calories attached. They mainly include the much drier grains and beans. We might call these the stars of nutrition – not as prestigious as the superstars, but winners nonetheless. Because they have less water and more calories, the foods in this group need to be eaten in somewhat smaller portions. If the superstars occupy half of your plate, the stars could be about one quarter.[72]

Also notice that grains and beans can move up and become superstars by simply cooking them. Cooking adds water, lowers the calorie count, and puts them in line for a significant promotion.

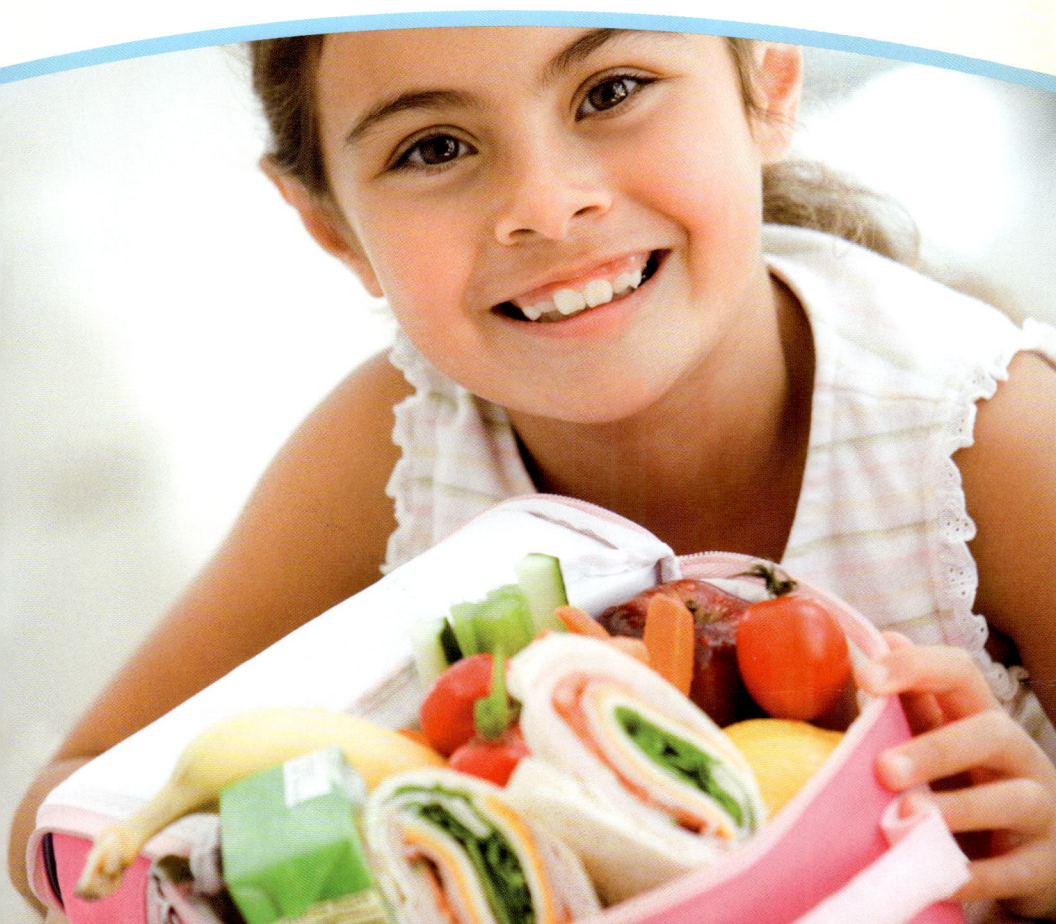

TINY CHOICES

In order to begin adding fiber-rich foods to our menus, we need to follow what

I call, "The Law of the Legos."

Legos are those little plastic blocks that snap together to build anything from a gas station to a condo. The blocks are only about an inch long. Other Lego shapes are even smaller. Each part by itself is not very impressive. But if you patiently put them together, one by one, you eventually create what's on the front of the box or whatever else your imagination dreams up.

I could reason that the process would go much faster if each piece was the size of a regular construction brick. Imagine putting a box of one hundred full-sized red bricks under the Christmas tree for your third grader. It'd still be sitting there by the time he or she graduated from high school. Too intimidating. Too difficult. Too time consuming. Only little, tiny pieces attract young users, keep them motivated, and get the job done.

There is a lesson here for us adults as we seek to build new eating habits. It is best to add just one small fiber food at a time, perhaps one every week or two. Think of each one as putting another Lego piece in place, slowly, patiently, at your own pace. Experiment. Chock what you don't like up to a learning experience and keep moving forward. Make it a fun adventure.

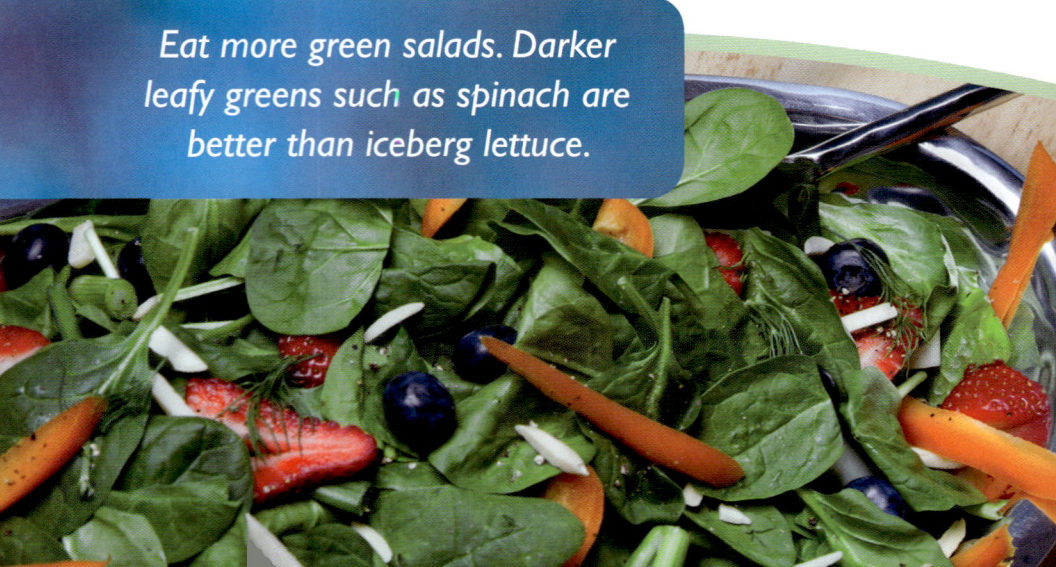

Eat more green salads. Darker leafy greens such as spinach are better than iceberg lettuce.

The following is a starter list of potential "Lego" pieces. Peruse the list, select one or two ideas that you like, add another later, and keep building over time.

- Eat more of the healthy foods you already like.
- Improve the quality of the foods you already enjoy. For instance, select a version with whole grains rather than refined grains, such as eating brown rice instead of white, rolled oatmeal instead of highly processed instant, or a bran muffin rather than chocolate chip.
- Utilize what the authors of *The Full Plate Diet* call "Power Ups." You simply add a high-fiber food to what you are already eating. For example, add fruit to your cereal, bananas to a peanut butter and jelly sandwich, or salsa atop a baked potato. Add or increase veggies in your fettuccine Alfred, lasagna, omelet, quesadilla, soups, pizza, spaghetti sauce, sandwich wrap, etc.[73]
- Eat more green salads. Darker leafy greens such as spinach are better than iceberg lettuce. Make it festive and colorful. Include tasty items such as chopped cucumbers, sliced zucchini, cherry tomatoes, onions, avocado, cranberries, raisins, shredded carrots, chopped nuts, radishes, red peppers, etc. Use an herb vinaigrette.[74] You can purchase bags of greens at the store to save time.
- Make more bean salads and fruit salads.
- Eat raw veggies with hummus or bean spread for snacks.
- Leave the skins on apples and potatoes.[75]
- Choose trail mix rather than a granola bar. Granola only has 1 gram of fiber, but trail mix with dried fruit has almost 3.[76]
- Exchange sweet potatoes for regular white potatoes.
- Eat a handful of nuts each day, such as walnuts or almonds.
- When you bake, substitute whole grain flour for half of the white flour.
- Use whole wheat pasta or mix with regular.
- Experiment with international dishes that use whole grains and legumes, such as Indian or Middle Eastern meals.[77]
- Make veggie stir fry or veggie kabobs.
- Replace white bread with a whole grain bread. If that is too drastic, make one slice whole grain and one slice white.

- Try split-pea soup.
- Sprinkle bran into your pancake mix.
- Bake an apple or pear rather than making a pie.[78]
- Eat an orange rather than drinking orange juice.
- When eating out, choose entrées that contain vegetables. Ask for extra veggies to be added.
- Order cooked vegetables on the side instead of fries.[79]
- Make fruit smoothies.
- Freeze grapes for a snack.
- Try a fruit you've never eaten before, such as a nectarine, plum, kiwifruit, papaya, pomegranate, kumquat, fig, date, blackberry, apricot, or mango.
- Keep fresh fruit in a visible place for snacks.
- If your children's favorite breakfast cereal is made from highly refined grains with too much sugar, help them slowly transition to a healthier option by pouring the entire box into a large bowl, mixing it with some portion of a whole grain cereal, and then putting it back in the original box. Get them to help you and ask them to give the new cereal a crazy name.
- Add one additional vegetable to one meal a week.
- Explore recipes that use garbanzo beans. See http://www.whfoods.com/genpage.php?tname=foodspice&dbid=58.

> Add fruit to your cereal, bananas to a peanut butter and jelly sandwich, or salsa atop a baked potato.

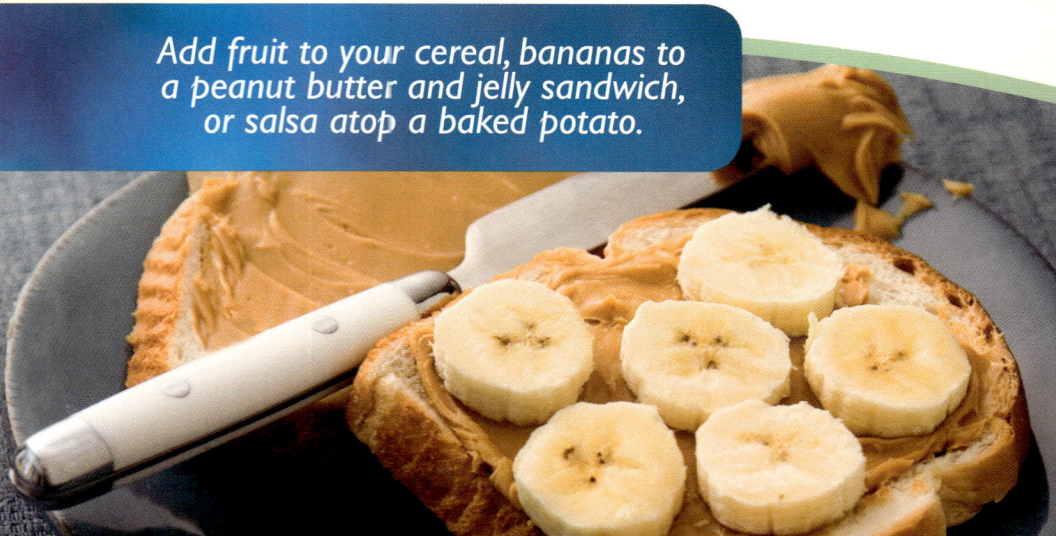

Good eating habits are formed one small choice at a time. It's as straightforward as reaching for an apple instead of potato chips. Tiny decisions add up and accumulate to become a healthier, happier you.

Making fiber-rich foods the centerpiece of eating has a long history. The Old Testament provides us with a remarkable story regarding their benefits. About six hundred years before Christ, the Israelite nation of Judah was attacked and defeated by a large army from the powerful country of Babylon.[80]

The Babylonians had a practice of taking the upper tier of people from a conquered nation and incorporating them into their own administration through a process of psychological, intellectual, and physical retraining.

Among the captives that were chosen for this reprogramming regimen were four of Israel's best young people named Daniel, Hananiah, Mishael, and Azariah. Far from home, at the mercy of their captives, it must have been a terrifying experience.

At mealtime, the king provided them with the rich foods of the well-to-do. Knowing the vital role that food plays in our physical and mental well-being, Daniel asked for vegetables instead. Their overseer was incredulous. He was convinced that such a simple diet would be totally inadequate and didn't dare make the switch. Daniel came up with the following proposal:

> "Please test your servants for ten days: Give us nothing but vegetables to eat and water to drink. Then compare our appearance with that of the young men who eat the royal food, and treat your servants in accordance with what you see." So he agreed to this and tested them for ten days. At the end of the ten days they looked healthier and better nourished than any of the young men who ate the royal food. So the guard took away their choice food and the wine they were to drink and gave them vegetables instead (Daniel 1:12–16, NIV).

> "Whenever the king consulted them in any matter requiring wisdom and balanced judgment, he found them ten times more capable than any of the magicians and enchanters in his entire kingdom" (Daniel 1:20, NLT).

The Bible could not have provided a more powerful endorsement!

RESOURCES:

If you are not used to cooking some of the fiber foods mentioned here and in the previous lesson, the following are some resources that can help:

BOOKS WITH RECIPES:

Simple Food For Busy Families, by Jeannette Bessinger and Tracee Yablon-Brenner

A Healthy Start: Energy Boosting Recipes and Tips, Tupperware and Florida Hospital Healthy 100

Vegetarian Cooking for Everyone, by Deborah Madison

Power Foods, From the Editors of Whole Living Magazine

Forks Over Knives, by Gene Stone

The Ultimate Volumetrics Diet, by Barbara Rolls

The Volumetrics Eating Plan, by Barbara Rolls

The Optimal Diet, by Hans Diehl and Darlene Blaney

Vegetarian Beginner's Guide, by Editors of Vegetarian Times

BOOKS WITHOUT RECIPES:

Full Plate Diet, by Stuart A. Seale, Teresa Sherard, and Diana Fleming. This best seller can be downloaded free as well as other resources at www.fullplateliving.org.

SuperSized Kids,
by Walt Larimore and Sherri Flynt

Becoming Vegetarian,
by Vesanto Melina and Brenda Davis

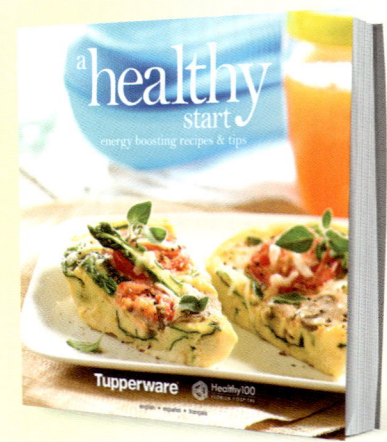

ONLINE VIDEOS ABOUT COOKING:
www.monkeysee.com/categories/4-food-and-drink

WEBSITES WITH RECIPES:
www.fullplateliving.org/diet/recipes

www.fruitsandveggiesmorematters.org/main-recipes

www.webmd.com/food-recipes/default.htm

www.webmd.com/food-recipes/healthy-recipe-finder?ps=5#

www.webmd.com/food-recipes/healthy-recipe-finder

www.simpledish.com/

www.recipe.com

www.supercook.com

www.choosemyplate.gov

www.epicurious.com (click on "Recipes & Menus" then select "healthy")

http://vegetarian.about.com/od/maindishentreerecipes/u/easyrecipes.htm

www.foodnetwork.com/healthy-every-week/package/index.html

www.webmd.com/diet/healthy-kitchen-11whole-grains-cooking?page=1

www.webmd.com/diet/healthy-kitchen-11/great-grains?page=1

www.webmd.com/diet/healthy-kitchen-11/best-cook-vegetables?page=1

www.eatingwell.com/healthy_cooking/healthy_cooking_101/shopping_cooking_guides/guide_to_cooking_20_vegetables

http://recipefinder.nal.usda.gov/

http://www.health.com/health/recipes/

http://www.cookinglight.com/food/vegetarian/

http://www.health.com/health/gallery/0,,20320446,00.html

http://www.cookinglight.com/food/quick-healthy/healthy-soup-recipes-00412000070018/

DISCUSSION

Was there a time in your life, or the life of someone you know, when there was too little food to eat? If so, describe.

....
....

In your own words, what distinction does the lesson make between "superstar" foods and "star" foods? Why is that important?

....
....

Was there anything that surprised you about how much water is in certain foods?

....
....

Which of the "Tiny Choices" did you find most appealing and doable? Why?

....
....

How many healthy snacks can the group describe?

....
....

Specifically, how could you add more fiber to one of your favorite recipes or foods this coming week?

....
....

How can you get more fiber when you eat out?

....
....

If you opened a fast food restaurant that only served high-fiber, low-fat foods, what would the menu be like?

....
....

SHARING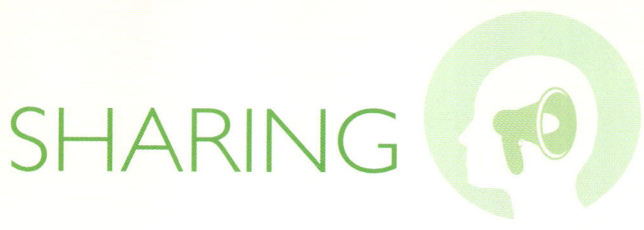

OPPORTUNITY #4:

- Pray for God to open the way for you to share something from these lessons to help someone else this week.
- Keep your radar up each day for opportunities.

ABUNDANT LIVING THOUGHT
Good eating habits are formed one small choice at a time.

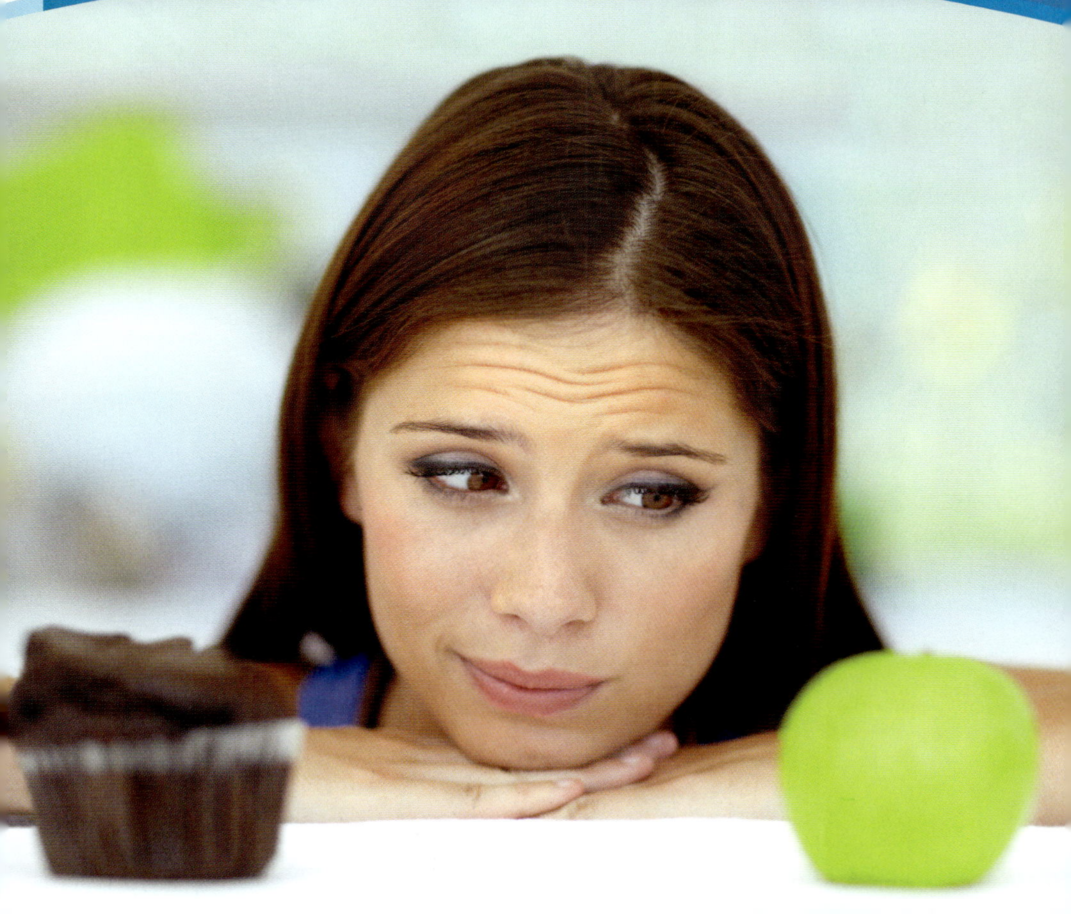

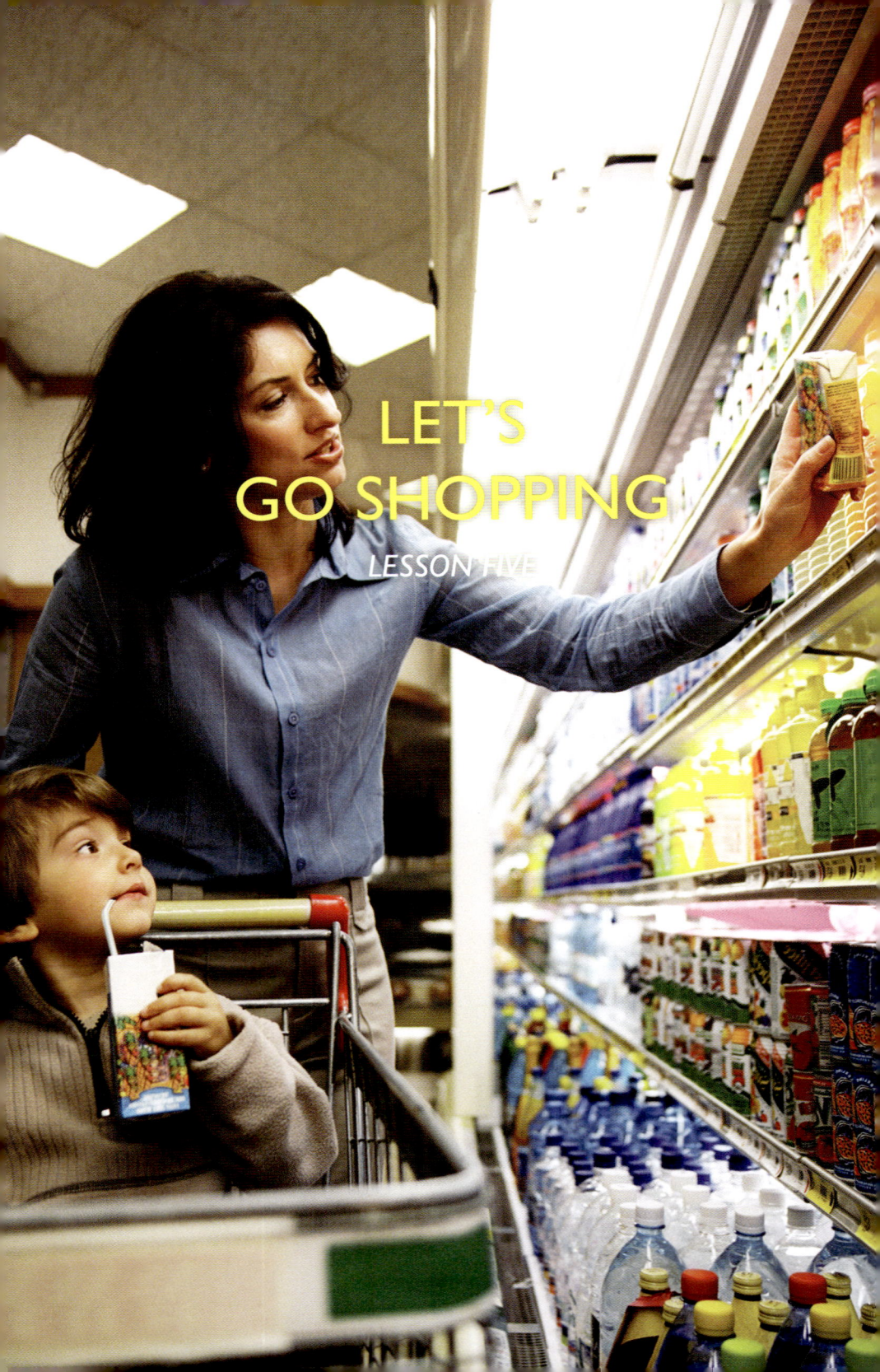

WARM UP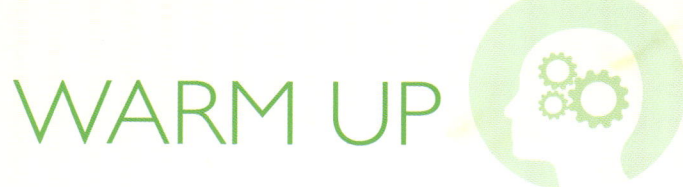

Feedback: In what ways did God open the door last week for you share some part of the lessons with someone else?

....
....
....
....

Choose one or both questions to discuss (if in group setting) or write out your answers on a separate sheet (for individual use):

1. **Who in the world would you like to job shadow?**[81]

....
....
....

2. **What makes you "come alive"?**[82]

....
....
....

> *"If it came from a plant, eat it; if it was made in a plant, don't."*
> **MICHAEL POLLAN**

DISCOVERY

About twenty years ago our car was on its last legs, so I decided to shop for a better used one. The main problem was that you never knew what you were getting. It was a real throw of the dice. Did the previous owner baby the car or abuse it?

I also hated negotiating the price. A friend told me about a strategy that was guaranteed to put the power back into the buyer's hands. You were supposed to give the salesperson your bottom line, and if they refused, you'd start to leave. Such a hard-nosed approach was supposed to bring the desperate salesperson to their knees.

I needed more power, so I adopted the plan. Firm-lipped, I strode into the dealer's office and was immediately met by a hefty man with a height advantage. I didn't mind because I had a plan.

He ushered me to his desk. "So, Mr. Johnson," he began, "how can we help you today?"

"Well," I said, "I need a car, maybe three or four years old. Under fifty thousand miles would be nice."

"Ok," he replied, leaning back. "I'm sure we can work that out. Any particular make and model?"

"Yeh, I was thinking about a Honda Civic." I gave him my offer.

"Ooo," he retorted, "that's kinda low. We'd go out of business at prices like that."

Time for the power. "Well," I told him, "I guess I'll have to look elsewhere." I got up, said my farewell, and started for the exit. Half way, I looked back and noticed he was smiling. At the exit I took one last glance, and he was still grinning. He even waved good-bye. As I stepped through the door, all of the power evaporated.

I'm still a terrible negotiator, but since those early days, there are now several online resources that have, thankfully, removed the uncertainty about what you're getting in a used car. You can find lots of information about the owner history, any accidents, maintenance record, type of usage, odometer reading, etc.

The same type of thing has happened when it comes to shopping for food. Buyers used to be at the mercy of the food industry. Manufacturers could make any claims they wanted to on the packaging, and the customer had no way of sorting out truth from hype, fact from fiction.

All that changed several years ago when the federal government required food manufacturers to put a "Nutrition Fact" label on every box and bag they produced. They specified exactly what information the label had to contain so that buyers could make good decisions. It was a tremendous win for the consumer.

This lesson will show you how to use that information to your best advantage. Such knowledge is indeed power and a big key to better nutrition and better health. You owe it to yourself and those you purchase food for to be informed.

Of course, foods purchased in the produce department don't need any label. But when it comes to manufactured foods, the Nutrition Facts label is absolutely vital.

In this lesson we'll briefly examine the food label from two perspectives:

1. How to understand it
2. How it can help you outwit the food industry

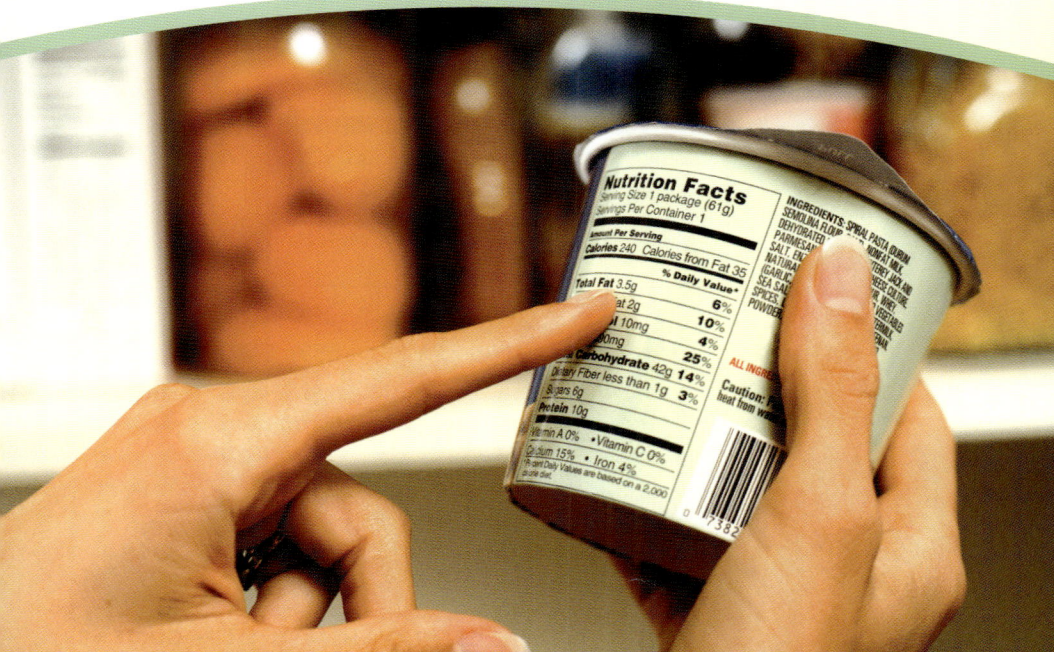

UNDERSTANDING THE NUTRITION FACTS LABEL

Entire books have been written on this topic, so we'll only be able to cover some of the main points. For further research, consult the Resources section at the end of this lesson.

Below is a sample label for some kind of food. *Don't get nervous about all the numbers. You only need to focus on a few things to know a lot.* The points are lettered for easy reference.

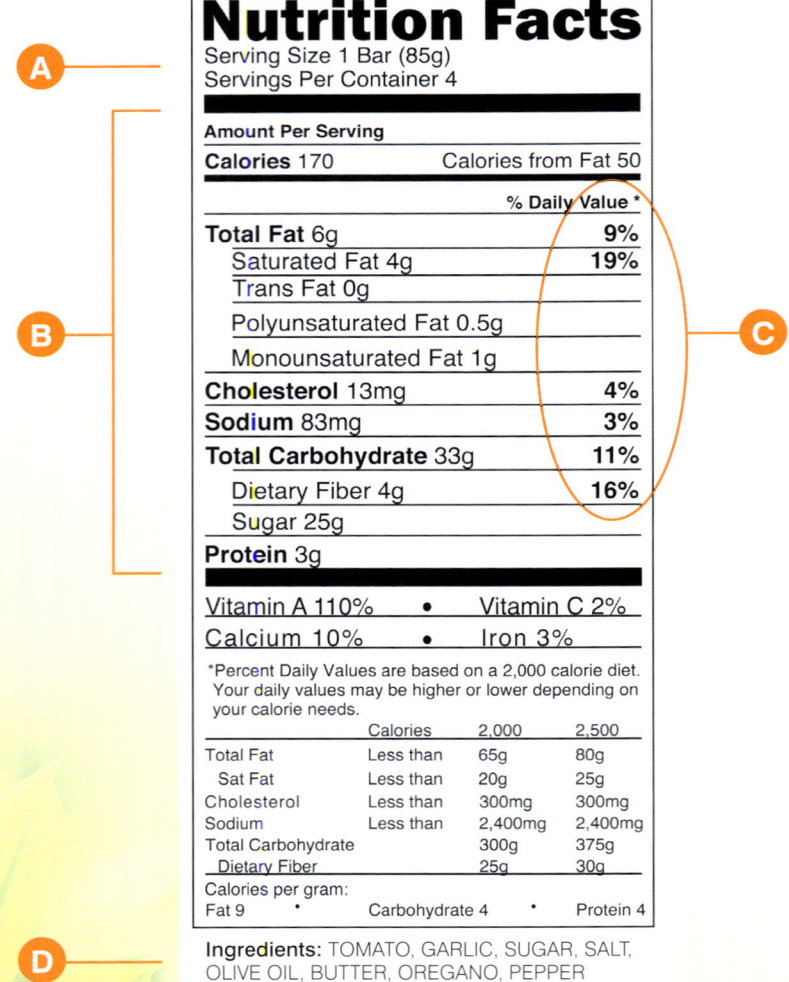

A – Serving Size. Section A of the label tells you the size of one serving. In this example it is ½ cup. It also tells you that there are supposed to be four servings in the package.

B – List Of Key Stats. The items in this list, from calories to protein, are the key factors affecting your health. The big point here is that the numbers right next to each item are based on *one serving only, not the entire package.*[83] So, in this example, if you happened to eat the entire contents, all of the numbers would have to be multiplied by four servings. For instance, total fat would go from one gram per serving to four grams for the entire package.

C – % Daily Value. The numbers on the right underneath the heading "% Daily Value" indicate what percentage you are getting of the recommended amount for an entire day. Use the following guideline:

Anything on the label that is 5 percent and under is a low amount, anything over 20 percent is a high amount, and anything in between is medium.[84]

This guideline applies to the good stuff and the bad. The best foods have lower percentages of total fat, cholesterol, and sodium, and a higher percentage of dietary fiber. Some items don't have officially recommended amounts.

The best way to compare different foods is to use the % Daily Value and Ingredients list for each one. Check to make sure the serving size is the same for each food.[85]

D – Ingredients. When you are looking at a Nutrition Facts label, this is the best place to start even though it is placed at the bottom. All of the ingredients in a product are named here. *It is important to understand that ingredients are listed in descending order according to weight.* This means that the largest amount is listed first and the smallest is listed last.[86]

The big point to remember is that *the first three ingredients usually tell the story of what you are getting.* Also, the fewer the number of ingredients the better.

Note that even though a product may have a lot of one healthy ingredient, it can be offset by another unhealthy one. *For instance, the benefits of high fiber can be offset by high sugar, fat, or salt.*

OUTWITTING THE FOOD INDUSTRY

Federal regulations don't always provide adequate safeguards for consumers as the food industry tries to find ways to maximize profits that are too often detrimental to our health. The following insights will give you the awareness you need to outwit the industry and come out ahead.

When Zero Isn't Zero

Fats merit careful attention because of the escalating incidence of heart disease alone. They are such a big deal that the Nutrition Facts label actually lists them according to type.

Not all fats are bad. Unsaturated fats, which include polyunsaturated and monounsaturated fats, are the good guys and can be eaten in moderation.[87]

Saturated fats, such as meat, butter, cheese, milk, and ice cream, are highest in animal products. They are not good for your heart, and their intake should be kept as low as possible.

Trans fats are the real bad boys of the health world. They should be completely eliminated from your diet. The food industry knows this, so they lobbied to be allowed to say a product has "zero" trans fats if it has half a gram (0.5) per serving or less. As a result, if there is half a gram in one serving and you happen to eat six servings, you actually get three grams of trans fat (0.5 X 6). Not good.

The way to tell if there really are zero trans fats or not is to look at the ingredients list. If you see the words "partially hydrogenated" or "vegetable shortening" anywhere, you can be sure there are trans fats hiding out.[88]

> *If someone buys a bag of cookies and the serving size is one cookie, what is the likelihood they will stop at one?*

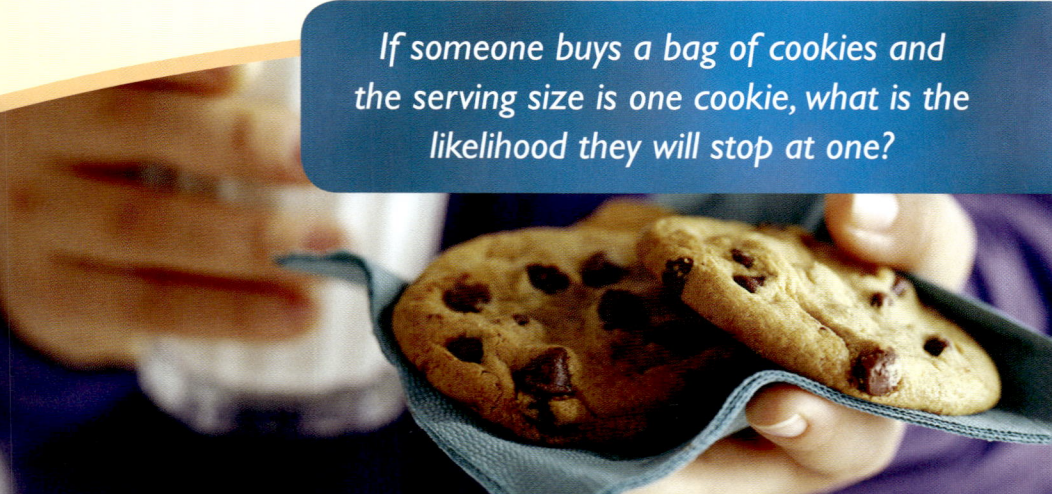

Ridiculous Serving Sizes

Another way some in the food industry try to skirt regulation is to lower the serving size to ridiculous amounts. Because the numbers on the Nutrition Facts label are *per serving,* the lower the serving size, the lower the numbers. Their goal is to get items like trans fats below the threshold where the numbers have to be reported. If someone buys a bag of cookies and the serving size is one cookie, what is the likelihood they will stop at one?[89]

Using Grainy Sounding Words

It is best to look for *whole grains* because they contain all three parts of the kernel – the germ, bran, and endosperm. Otherwise you will be missing some vital nutrients.

The food industry often chops the grain up and uses only the starchy inside because it lasts longer on the shelf. The problem is that most of the great nutrition is in what they took away. Out of the goodness of their hearts they add back a handful of lost nutrients and call it "enriched." Would you feel enriched if someone stole $100 and gave you back $2? I don't think so! Examples of enriched foods include favorites like white bread and white rice – fattening and not very nourishing.[90]

To get you to think you are getting the whole grain when you aren't, the food industry uses a lot of "grainy sounding words" in their marketing and in the ingredients list. Foods with the following words on the label are not 100% whole-grain – "100% wheat, multi-grain, seven grains."[91] Manufacturers also try to make you think a food is whole grain by using brown coloring such as molasses.

The only way to know you are getting the entire grain is to look on the ingredients list for the magic word "whole" followed by the name of the grain, such as "100% whole wheat, whole wheat, or whole grain wheat."

And make sure it is the very first item on the Nutrition Facts ingredients list. Because the list has the largest amounts first, the second ingredient could be anywhere from 49 percent to as little as 1 percent.

To get foods with healthy amounts of whole grain, a good rule of thumb is look for three to five grams of fiber.[92]

Making Sugars Hard to Find

It is very important to pay attention to sugar on the Nutrition Facts label because obesity and diabetes have skyrocketed in recent years. Heart disease has also been implicated.[93] Scientists have even discovered that sugar can, in fact, be addictive.[94]

Manufacturers add sugars to tens of thousands of foods during processing.[95] About four grams of sugar equal one teaspoon, and it is recommended that women eat no more than six teaspoons of added sugar each day, and nine teaspoons for men.[96] The Centers for Disease Control reports that the average person in the US consumes *over twenty-seven teaspoons of added sugar every day.*[97]

We get most of it in sodas, sports drinks, fruit drinks, and energy drinks. Just one twelve-ounce can of cola has almost ten teaspoons of sugar, and cranberry juice cocktail has over eleven. The Center for Science in the Public Interest calls these drinks "liquid candy."[98] Added sugars are also in lots of other products from tomato sauce and bread to baby food.

The Nutrition Facts label lists the grams of sugar per serving. The ingredients list also provides valuable information about how much sugar you are getting. If sugar is one of the first three ingredients, treat it like a dessert to be eaten sparingly or avoided entirely.

Food manufacturers know that smart shoppers are turned off when sugar appears high up on the ingredients list, so they have *devised a clever strategy to get around that issue.* They simply use several different added sugars in smaller amounts so they show up much farther down the ingredients list, scattered among other items. You may not recognize them because they have unfamiliar names. But you can spot them if you know what to look for.

> *The average person in the US consumes over twenty-seven teaspoons of added sugar every day. We get most of it in sodas, sports drinks, fruit drinks, and energy drinks.*

Here are some of the sugars that can be added during processing.[99] The most common one is high fructose corn syrup.

- Brown sugar
- Cane sugar
- Corn sweetener
- Corn syrup
- Dextrose
- Fructose
- Glucose
- High-fructose corn syrup
- Malt syrup

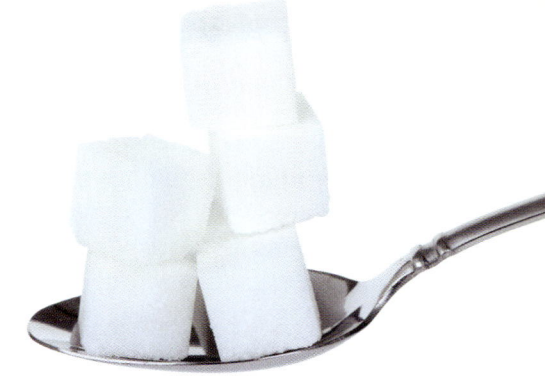

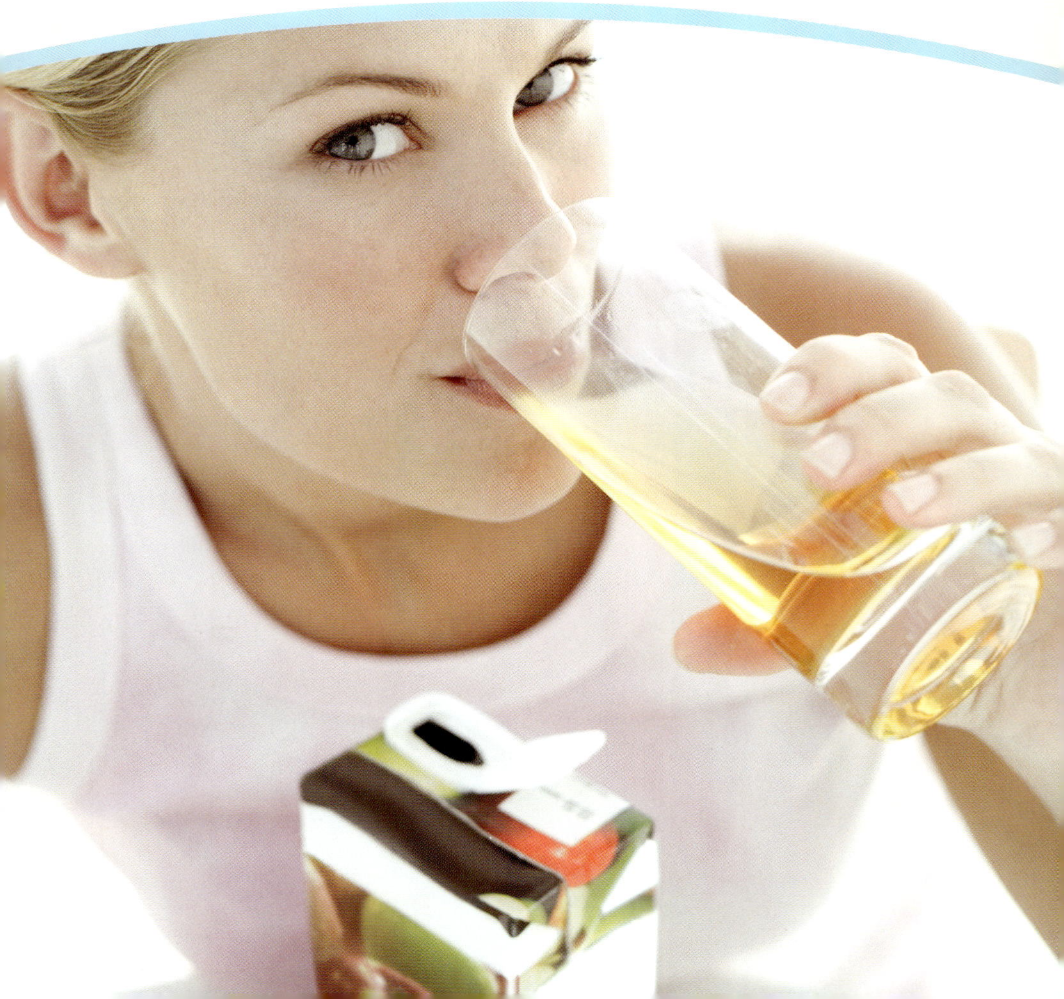

Other Names for Sodium

Excess salt is another bandit robbing us of health. Excess consumption of sodium raises blood pressure and is a major player in stroke, heart disease, and heart attacks. The average American gets more than twice the American Heart Association recommendation of 1,500 mg per day.[100]

Over 75 percent of our sodium intake comes from processed foods or restaurant meals rather than the salt we add ourselves. So watch the Nutrition Facts label % Daily Value at the grocery store. Also check out the ingredients list. Sodium can show up under various names such as: monosodium glutamate, sodium citrate, sodium nitrate, sodium phosphate, sodium saccharin, and also as baking soda or baking powder in baked goods.[101]

Thankfully there is a promise in Scripture of special assistance from God when we are faced with confusing decisions in all the various areas of life, which includes what we eat. In the New Testament book of James we read, "If any of you lacks wisdom, you should ask God, who gives generously to all" (James 1:5, NIV). He cares about our food choices and is eager to help.

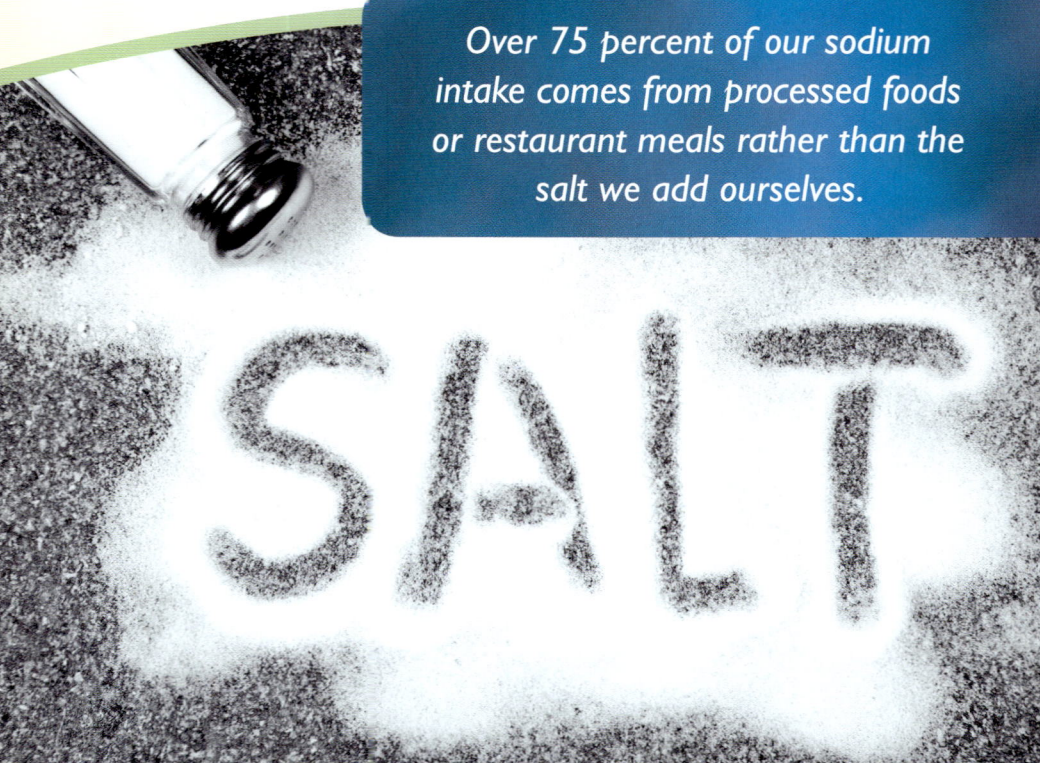

Over 75 percent of our sodium intake comes from processed foods or restaurant meals rather than the salt we add ourselves.

Resources On Nutrition Facts Labels:
www.kidshealth.org/parent/nutrition_center/healthy_eating/food_labels.html#

www.fda.gov/Food/ResourcesForYou/Consumers/ucm266853.htm

Resources For General Nutrition Information:
www.nutrition.gov/

www.choosemyplate.gov/

www.letsmove.gov/

www.eatright.org/Public/

www.eatright.org/Shop/Product.aspx?id=6442473967
Pocket Supermarket Guide, Academy of Nutrition and Dietetics
[Need to purchase. Excellent.]

www.hsph.harvard.edu/nutritionsource/

www.nutrition411.com/

www.webmd.com/food-recipes/default.htm

www.mayoclinic.com/health/HealthyLivingIndex/HealthyLivingIndex

www.todaysdietitian.com/

www.cnpp.usda.gov/dietaryguidelines.htm

www.diabetes.org

www.americanheart.org

www.wholegrainscouncil.org

www.fda.gov/food/default.htm

www.fns.usda.gov

www.nhlbi.nih.gov/health/public/heart/obesity/lose_wt/lcal_fat.htm

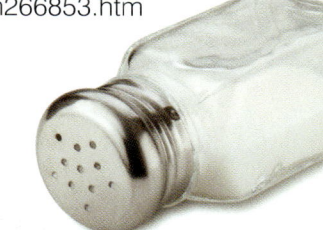

DISCUSSION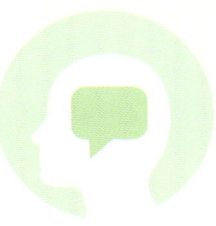

Have the group discuss the four key aspects of the Nutrition Facts label covered in the lesson (A,B,C,D).

....
....

What is the most helpful insight you gained from learning about the Nutrition Facts label?

....
....

What are some of your greatest challenges in figuring out whether processed foods are healthy or not?

....
....

What is good or bad about each of these ingredients lists from Nutrition Facts labels?

1. Whole grain oats, corn starch, sugar, salt, tripotassium phosphate, wheat starch, vitamin E.

   ....
   ....

2. Rice, whole wheat, sugar, whole oats, wheat bran, strawberry-flavored apple pieces, modified palm kernel oil, corn syrup, salt, brown sugar syrup, modified milk ingredients, brown sugar, barley malt syrup, rice flour, vegetable oil, polydextrose, monoglycerides, tapioca dextrin.

   ....
   ....

3. Tomato puree, diced tomatoes, sugar, dehydrated garlic, salt, dried onions, extra virgin olive oil, oregano, celery powder, citric acid, marjoram.

   ....
   ....

SHARING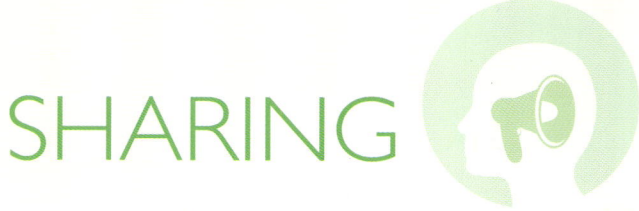

OPPORTUNITY #5:

- Pray for God to open the way for you to share something from these lessons to help someone else this week.
- Keep your radar up each day for opportunities.

ABUNDANT LIVING THOUGHT

The big point to remember is that the first three ingredients usually tell the story of what you are getting.

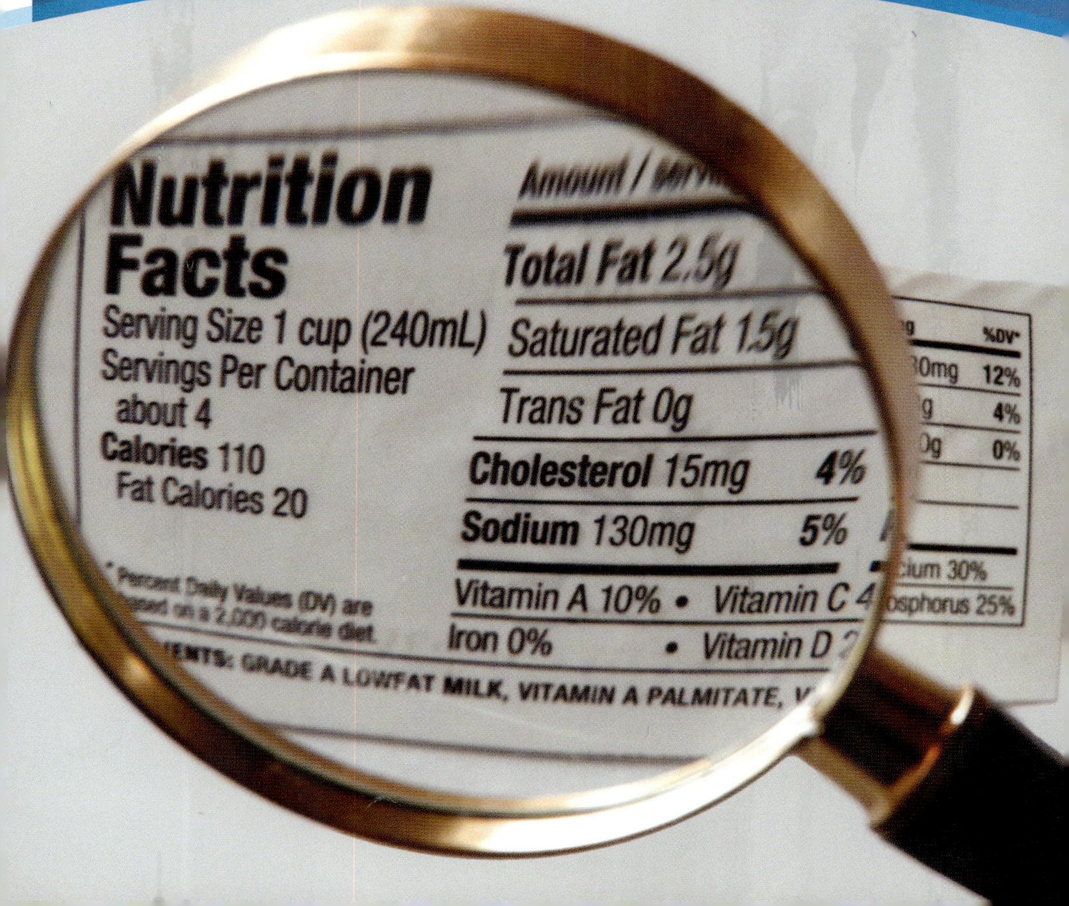

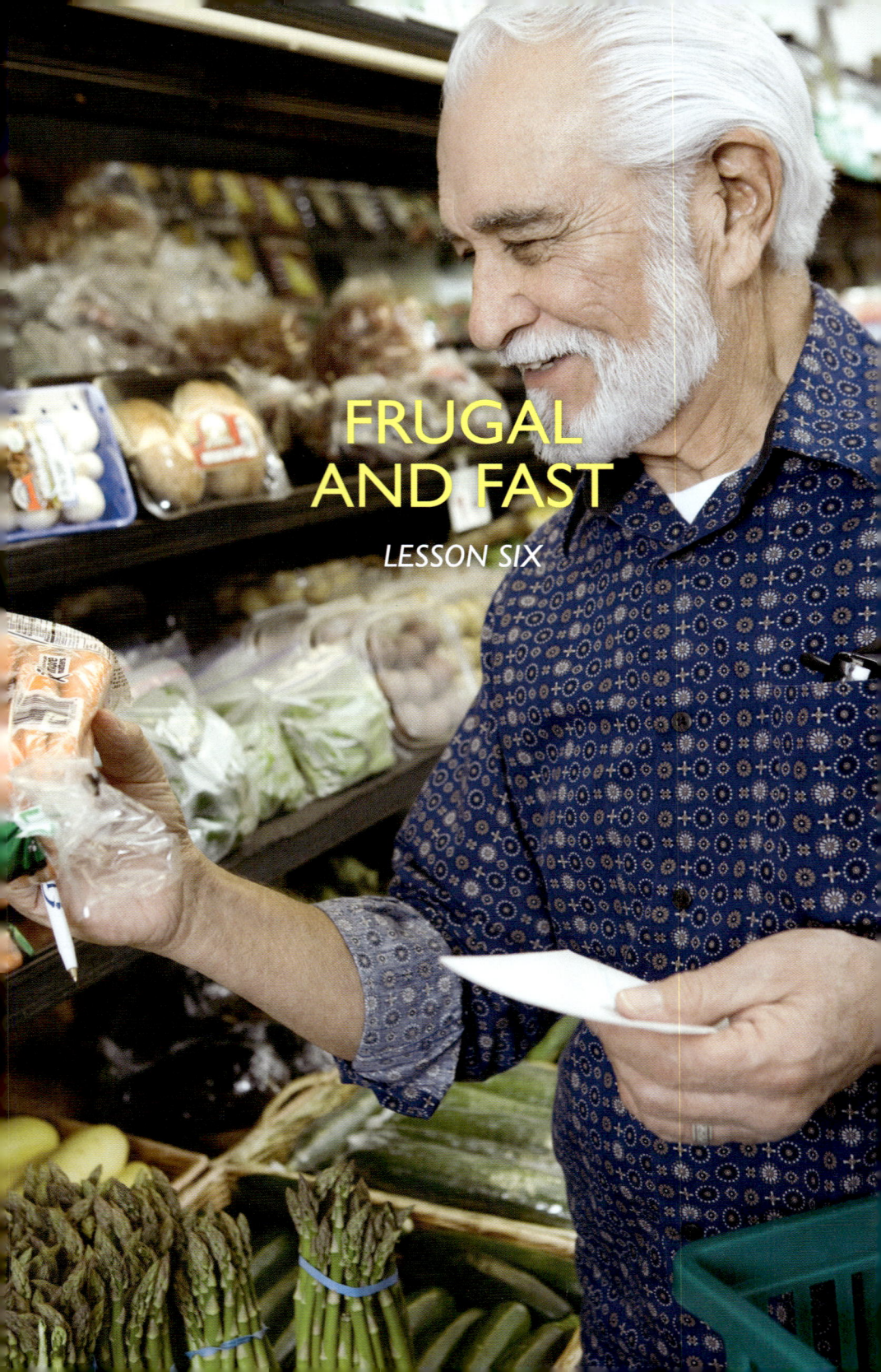

FRUGAL AND FAST

LESSON SIX

WARM UP

Feedback: In what ways did God open the door last week for you share some part of the lesson with someone else?

....
....
....
....

Choose one or both questions to discuss (if in group setting) or write out your answers on a separate sheet (for individual use):

1. **Tell something about yourself that no one in the group probably knows.**[102]

....
....
....

2. **What did you like most about the best boss you ever had?**[103]

....
....
....

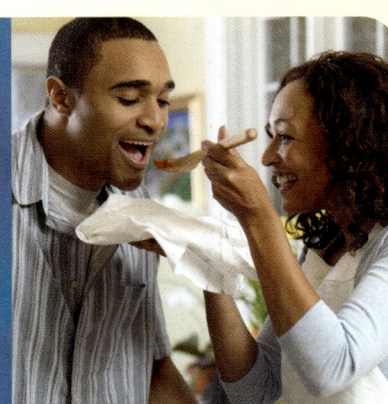

"This is my invariable advice to people: learn how to cook. Try new recipes, learn from your mistakes, be fearless, and above all have fun!"

JULIA CHILD

CREATION HEALTH | LIFE GUIDE #8

DISCOVERY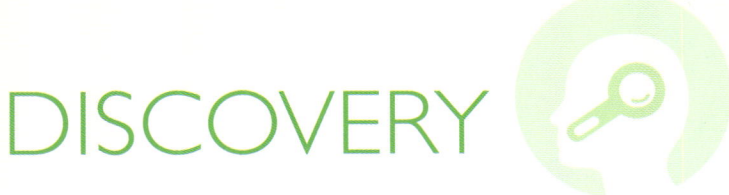

When I look at the index finger of my right hand, my mind is sometimes carried back to my high school days when I worked in a supermarket. I started out as a bag boy and eventually graduated to checkout clerk. This was the old days – before scanners – when you had to actually push buttons on a cash register and make crucial decisions like whether or not something was taxable.

From there I entered the mysterious back room world of produce – cutting, weighing, measuring, wrapping, engineering displays. After earning my stripes at that assignment, I finally arrived at what I considered the pinnacle of supermarket life – stock boy in the main aisles. It was exhilarating to work with veteran stockers. I was even assigned my own cutter. That's where my right index finger enters the picture.

One day I was opening a series of cardboard boxes with my razor-sharp cutter. I had learned how to turn the box with one hand while simultaneously cutting the top edge with the other. It was poetry in motion. On box number five, I got distracted, my index finger drooped below the edge, and . . . deep slice on the inside just above the first knuckle. Scar #1.

About a month later, the same thing happened again, same wayward finger, similar slice, but at more of an artsy angle. Scar #2.

As I worked those aisles day and night, I had no idea how carefully the entire store had been laid out by specialists in marketing psychology from headquarters. I have since learned that everything is thought through and positioned for one overriding purpose – to get us to spend more money. I don't blame the owners for wanting to maximize profits, but before I knew the plan I used to innocently stumble into their web and wind up shelling out too many dollars in the process.

First they usually force you to turn toward the bakery. This is why it is crucial to not shop when you are hungry. The smell reaches out, inviting you to linger and check out the great tasting, colorfully decorated sweets. The longer you linger anywhere in the store, the more you're likely to spend from impulse.[104]

Where I shop, you then hang a left and wind up in the deli. The salivary glands are now fully engaged, shouting at you, "I need!"[105]

Straight ahead is the produce department. It's positioned there to create warm, Mother Earth feelings that managers hope will carry over into other departments. This is the healthiest, safest place in the entire store. If you are going to linger anywhere, do it here. This is where to get the greatest bang for your hard-earned buck.

In our store the fruit-flavored beverages are located nearby, lined up along several large shelves. The store designer wants you to make a mental connection with produce and think that these drinks are as healthy as the whole fruit. The truth is that most of them are loaded with sugar.

Have you noticed how they put the staples like bread and milk at the back of the store? That's to get you to wander through as much territory as possible before getting there. They also put the priciest items on the shelves at eye level. Manufacturers pay good money for that location. The less expensive store brands and bulk items are down below.

Other lures and enticements abound. The most profitable area for grocers is the checkout because that is where you wait the longest. There is a tantalizing lineup of magazines, candies, and bins where you can buy ten of something for only $4.99. Take a deep breath and resist.

Don't be uptight when you go grocery shopping; just be alert and wise.

The goal is to be a more aware, intentional shopper. To help you do that, this lesson contains some practical ways to save *money* on your food budget. We'll also look at how to save *time* shopping and preparing meals. The aim is to help you be both frugal and fast.

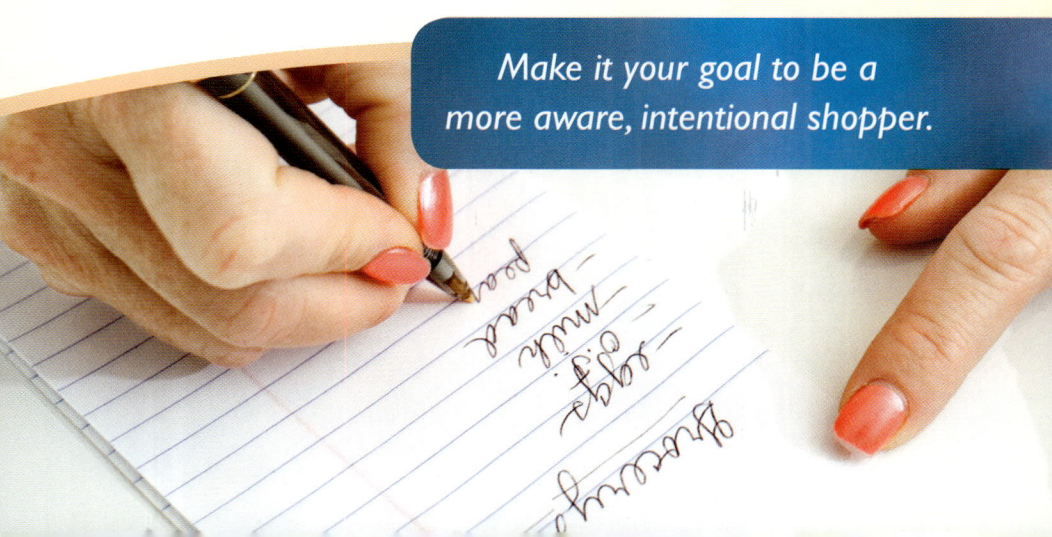

Make it your goal to be a more aware, intentional shopper.

SAVING MONEY

1. **Determine how much you are currently spending on food.**
You won't know where you can save unless you know how much you spend. Start by listing what food items you purchased over the last couple of weeks. Use your bank statements or actual receipts. Receipts can help you sort out grocery items you purchased at stores other than the supermarket. Don't forget cash payments, and be sure to include eating out. Group the expenses into various categories that you find meaningful.

2. **List specific cost-cutting measures.**
Look over your categories and select one or two items where immediate savings might occur. You can expand the list of cost savings over time. Too much change at once will cause pushback and discontent. If you have a family, this is a good time for collaboration and brainstorming so everyone is on the same page with no surprises.

3. **Picture what you'll do with the savings.**
Write down the projected savings and figure out what you'll do with the money. Simply "reducing expenses" is not as motivating as a tangible reward. It may be something small like buying a bouquet of flowers or something larger like a trip to the mall or saving for a vacation. Form a mental image of the reward actually happening in order to stay motivated when temptations to overspend arrive, as they surely will.[106]

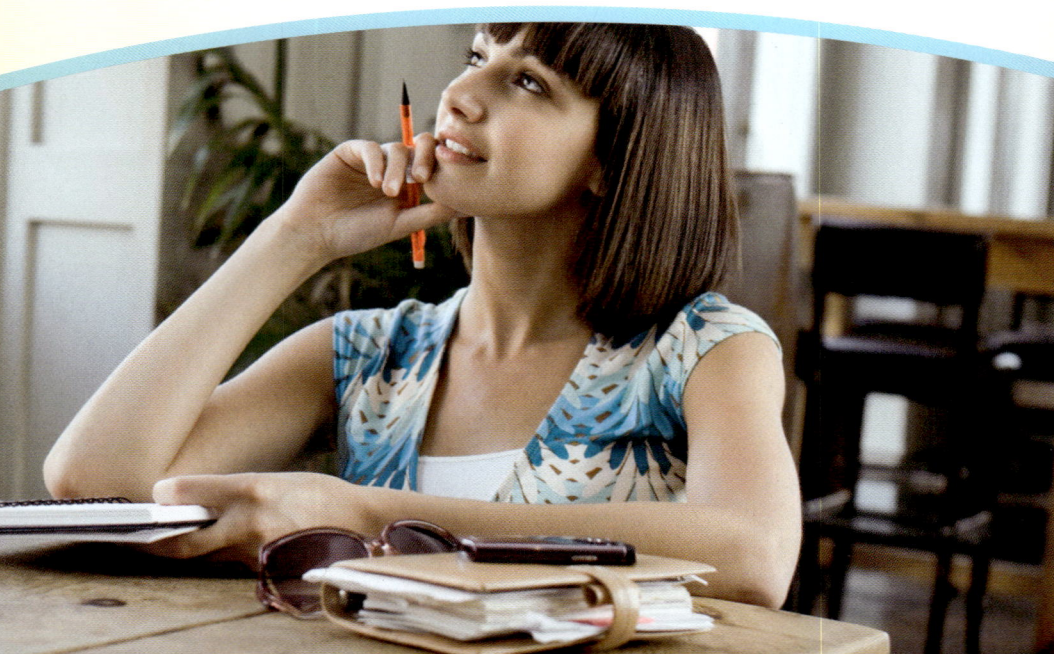

For example, you might decide that the family will eat out one less time a month, which could save $35. You can probably eat at home for less than half that amount, so there is a net savings of about $18. Three or four weeks like that, and you have a new pair of shoes! Rather than thinking of frugality as being restrictive, think of it as freeing up more options in your life.

4. Plan your meals.
Planning your meals is a major key to effective shopping because it puts you in control. To get in the habit, start by planning only the meals you already know how to cook. You can add more later. Write down all of the ingredients for each one. Focus mainly on the evening meal and lunches. You don't usually have to plan breakfast because many people eat basically the same thing each morning. Don't forget to consult the appointment calendar for you and the family. You don't want to fix a meal for four when two will be away at some activity.[107]

5. Make a shopping list.
There is a difference between a traditional shopping list and a "money saving" shopping list. The first simply repeats what you've done in the past. The second is forward looking and incorporates whatever cost-cutting measures you choose to implement.

Many people find it helpful to create an overall *Master Grocery List* of all the items they *might* purchase with no amounts specified.[108] You can write it out longhand and photocopy it, or you can create a spreadsheet and print copies each time you shop. This saves having to make a new list from scratch each week. It also serves as a reminder of what to consider.

A copy of the Master Grocery List then becomes a customized *Shopping List* each week. Simply put a check mark next to the items that you plan to buy and the amount, and then use the completed list when you go to the store. Be sure to do an inventory ahead of time to see what ingredients you already have on hand. It can be helpful to leave the list up on the refrigerator all week so people can mark an item when they think of it.

If you want to be an advanced shopper, include the prices next to as many items on your Master Grocery List as you can.[109] This way you can instantly tell if something is a good buy or not. You just have to make sure the sizes are the same.

The most accurate way to compare prices even if items are different sizes is to record what is called the "cost per unit."[110] The cost per unit is simply the price divided by the amount in whatever units it comes in – ounces, pounds, etc. For instance, if an item costs $8.00 and weighs eight ounces, the cost per ounce is $1.00 ($8.00 divided by eight ounces).

Bring a calculator to the store for quick checks. Many price tags on the shelves will do the cost per unit math for you. You can update the prices on your Master Grocery List as needed.

For some sample Master Grocery Lists, go to: http://www.grocerylists.org/ultimatest/.

6. Purchase fruits and vegetables in season.

Check with your produce manager to find out when various fruits and vegetables are in season. They are usually less expensive at that time. You can use savings in one area of the food budget to purchase healthier foods like this in another. Frozen is a good alternative and may cost less. Canned is also nutritious, but be careful regarding heavy syrup in canned fruits and too much sodium in canned veggies. The sodium can be significantly reduced by rinsing the contents.

7. Eat fewer empty calories.

Katherine Tallmadge, RD, author of the book *Diet Simple*, writes, "When my clients start eating more healthfully, their grocery bills plummet."[111] People can spend a lot of money on foods that are high in calories but low in nutritional value. These low-fiber foods don't satisfy their hunger for long, and so they wind up snacking way too much on expensive products.

8. Eat less meat or cut it out entirely.

Cutting back on meat consumption or eliminating it entirely is good for both your health and your wallet. If you eat meat, make it a side dish rather than the main feature. Also plan some meatless meals. There are lots of great, less-expensive vegetarian recipes available.[112]

More and more people are choosing a vegetarian lifestyle. If you do, don't worry about getting enough protein. Fiber-rich foods contain all of the protein you'll need. The United States Department of Agriculture states, "Protein needs can easily be met by eating a variety of plant-based foods."[113] Make the transition slowly by gradually serving smaller portions of meat and introducing delicious meatless meals over time.

SAVING TIME

1. **Shop as seldom as possible.**

If you plan meals for one week, try to go to the store only once a week. There are two reasons: (1) a lot of impulse buying occurs when people only intend to pop in for one or two items, and (2) it saves you time.

If you really want to save time, plan meals for more weeks. If you plan meals for two weeks, shop only once every two weeks.

2. **Prepare several meals at one time.**[114]

One of the reasons that people eat out so much is because they don't feel they have time to cook at home. To reduce time in the kitchen, try doing as much preparation as possible for the entire week's meals *at one time* rather than doing it every day. Cutting and chopping the same items for different recipes on one occasion is more efficient. Group the items for each meal in large Ziploc® plastic bags, label them with a magic marker, and put them in the freezer. Those who are more adventurous might even try working on two weeks of meals at a time. You may also be able to do cooking for more than one meal at a time. Doubling some recipes also saves effort by freezing each half.

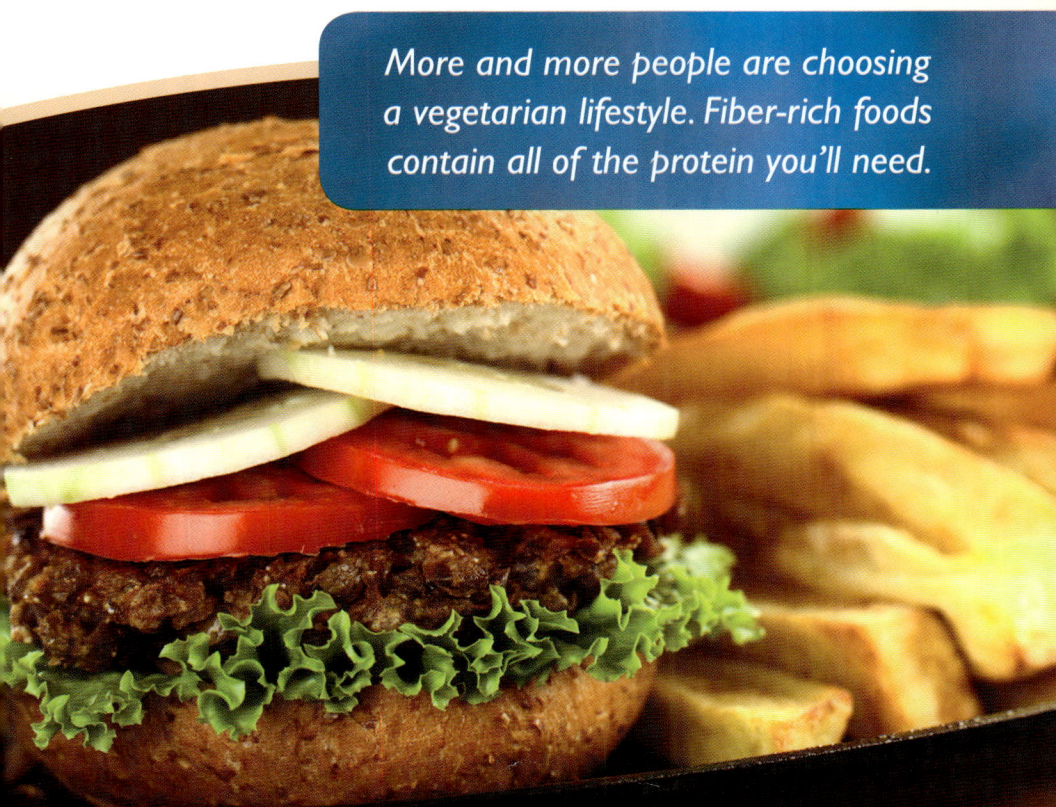

More and more people are choosing a vegetarian lifestyle. Fiber-rich foods contain all of the protein you'll need.

3. Prepare only one meal for everyone.
Sometimes parents become short-order cooks, making different meals each evening to accommodate different people's tastes. Such an approach wastes both time and money. You should be able to cook only one meal for everyone, especially if you involve others in meal planning.[115]

4. Get the family involved.
You will get more cooperation and save time if you involve the entire family in meal preparation. Little kids can set the table or put d shes in the dishwasher. Older children can do chopping and mixing. Teenagers can prepare the entire meal, especially if it is one of their choosing. Teaching children the skills of smart shopping and effective meal preparation is something they will have for the rest of their lives. Make it an adventure with lots of dialogue and laughter.

5. Consider using a crock pot/slow cooker.
You can place the ingredients inside in the morning and have it ready when you come home at night.

6. Choose recipes with only a few ingredients.
There are number of books and online resources that bring together healthy recipes with only a few ingredients with less preparation time such as those listed below.

In the Old Testament book of Isaiah we read, "Why spend your money on food that does not give you strength? Why pay for food that does you no good? Listen to me, and you will eat what is good. You will enjoy the finest food" (Isaiah 55:2, NLT). Eating the healthiest foods doesn't happen by chance. It comes from listening to God's guidance and seeking to increase our awareness and planning. Those qualities will take what you eat to a whole new level and put you squarely in charge of the role food plays in your life.

Resources to save money:
Cut Your Grocery Bill In Half, Steve and Annette Economides

Family Feasts for $75 a Week, Mary Ostyn

Healthy Meals for Less, Jonni McCoy

Eat Cheap but Eat Well, Charles Mattocks

Money Smart Family website: www.moneysmartfamily.com/

Resources to save time:
Simple Food for Busy Families, Jeannette Bessinger and Tracee Yablon-Brenner

Resources - General
A Healthy Start, Tupperware Cooking Collection

Eat This Not That: Supermarket Survival Guide, David Zinczenko

Eat This Not That: Kitchen Survival Guide, David Zinczenko

Becoming Vegetarian, Vesanto Melina and Brenda Davis

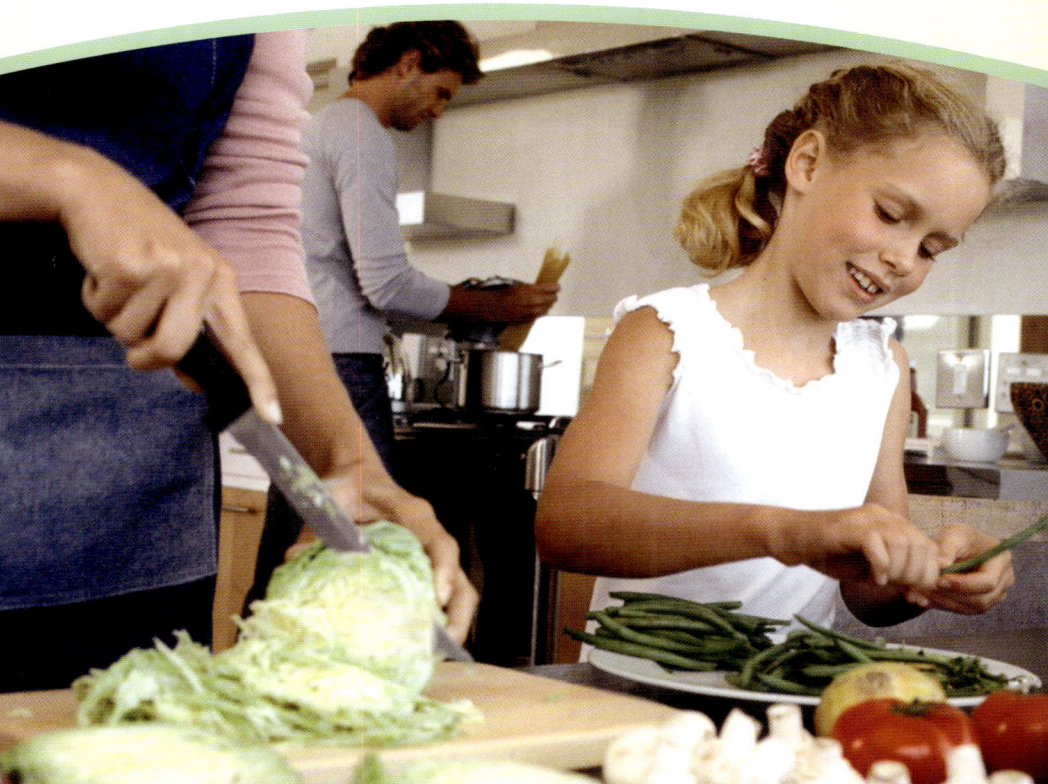

DISCUSSION

What ideas do you have about how to save on the food budget in addition to those in this lesson?
....
....

How did you learn how to cook? What were some of the most helpful ideas you have picked up?
....
....

What sources do you use to find great recipes?
....
....

What are your biggest challenges in developing a shopping list? What can help?
....
....

What methods have you found most effective for saving time preparing meals?
....
....

Share one of your favorite meals that takes under thirty minutes to prepare.
....
....

How would you go about fixing several days meals at one time?
....
....

What are some practical ways to get children more involved in meal preparation?
....
....

SHARING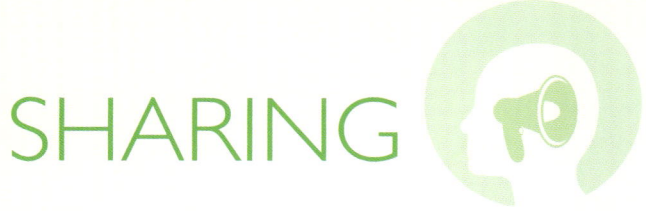

OPPORTUNITY #6:

- Pray for God to open the way for you to share something from these lessons to help someone else this week.
- Keep your radar up each day for opportunities.

ABUNDANT LIVING THOUGHT

Planning your meals is a major key to effective shopping because it puts you in control.

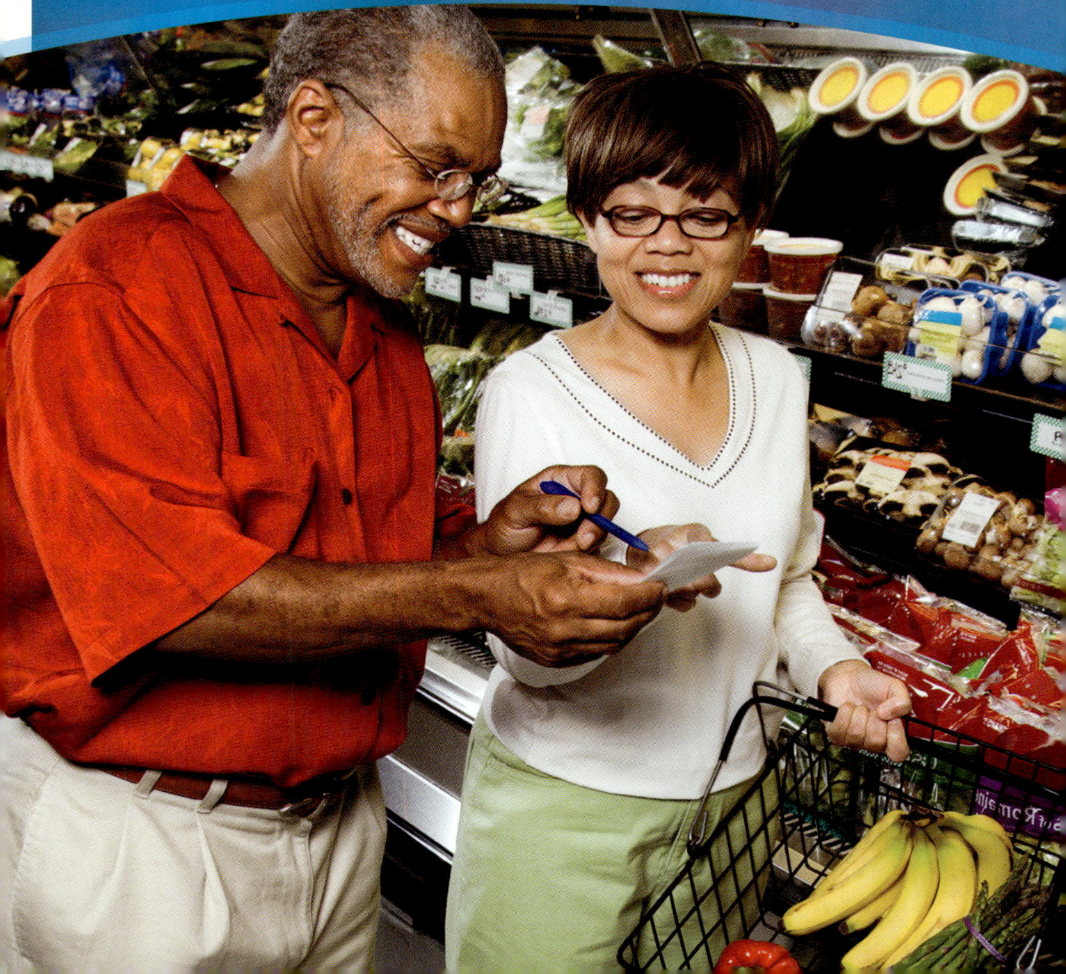

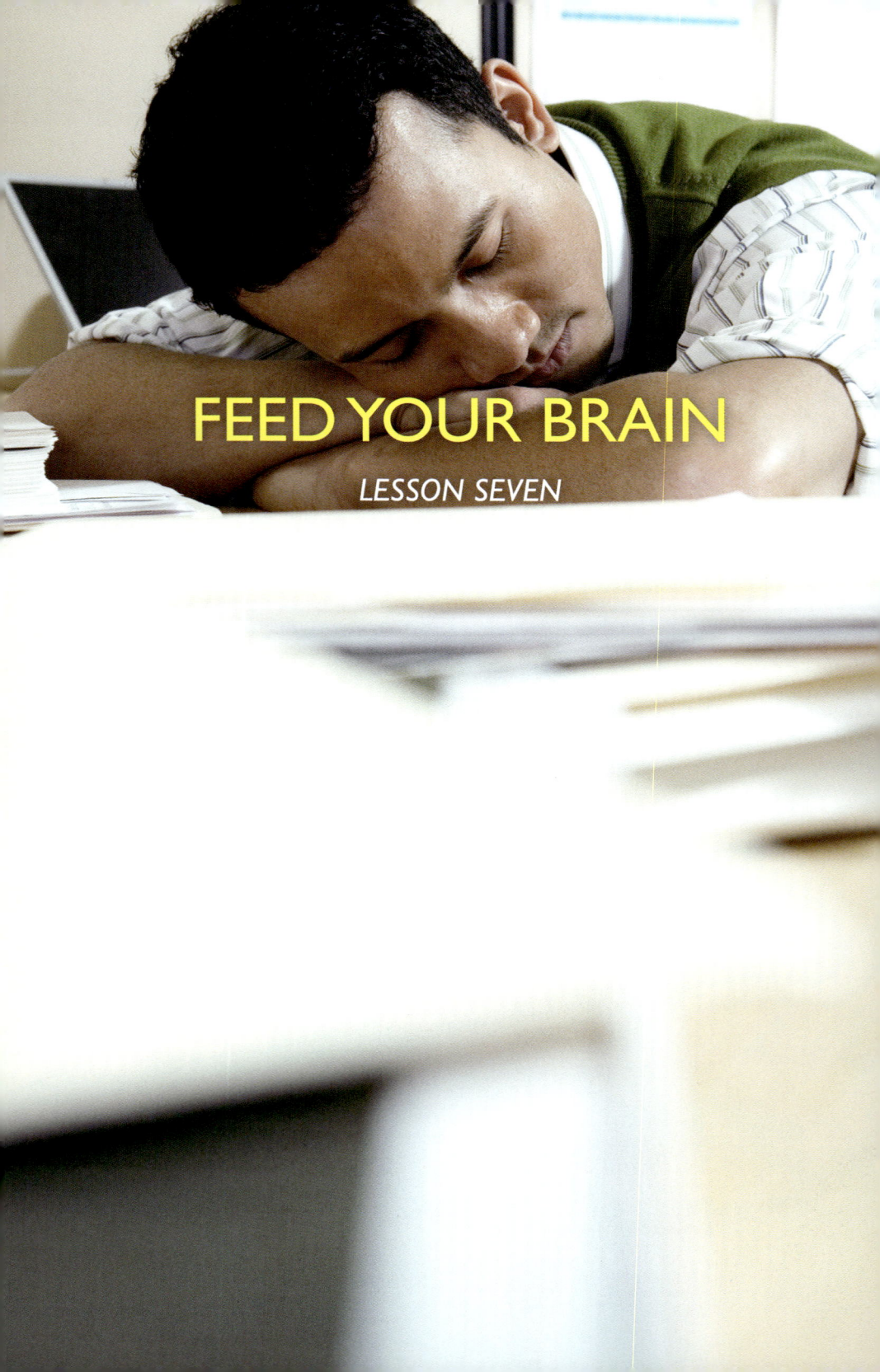

FEED YOUR BRAIN

LESSON SEVEN

WARM UP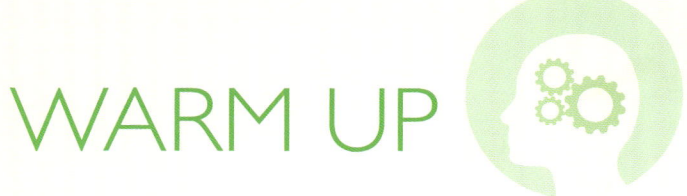

Feedback: In what ways did God open the door last week for you share some part of the lessons with someone else?

....
....
....

Choose one or both questions to discuss (if in group setting) or write out your answers on a separate sheet (for individual use):

1. **Tell about one of the best phone calls you ever received.**[116]

....
....
....

2. **One of the most difficult things to learn in life is ...**[117]

....
....
....

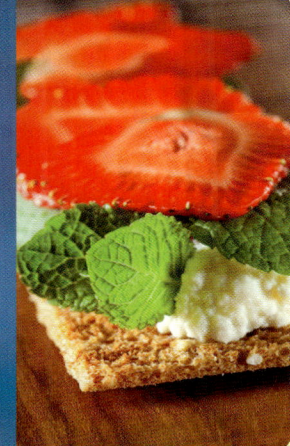

"It should come as no surprise that eating a balanced diet with plenty of fruits, vegetables, grains, and dairy products that reduce your risk of heart attacks would also help with keeping your brain in top condition."

MAJID FOTUHI, MD, PhD

DISCOVERY

As the American Airlines jet approached Reagan National Airport in Washington, DC, on Wednesday, March 23, 2011, the pilot felt increasingly frustrated and bewildered. He checked the time. It was ten minutes after midnight. He had just been in contact with the controller at the regional facility in Warrenton, VA, for the last fifty miles of the uneventful trip from Dallas, TX. Now that the plane was within five miles of the airport and under 2,500 feet, it was supposed to be handed off to the local tower to get the final information on wind speed, area traffic, and clearance to land. Reagan tower, however, was unresponsive.

The pilot called Reagan again, but still no reply. He stared into the night, wondering what to do next. As the 737 sped closer to its final destination, the pilot knew he had to make a decision quickly. With ninety-one people on board, he chose to abort the landing and give himself time to think.

The only option was to get back in touch with the regional facility he had just signed off from. The controller there said he also had not been able to make contact with the tower, even after using a landline. The decision was made to go ahead and land anyway with the regional controller providing guidance the entire way.

Gripping the controls a little more tightly than usual and studying the ground ahead intently, the American Airlines pilot brought the plane in for a safe landing.

Fifteen minutes later, a United Airlines Airbus 320 from Chicago ran into the same disturbing problem. He too relied on the regional office and landed without incident.

The small number of flights at that early hour lowered the risk to an acceptable level. If the incident had happened at a busier time of day, the potential of hitting another plane taxiing across the runway would have ratcheted up the danger enormously.

During a later investigation, the unavailable controller at Reagan revealed that he had actually fallen asleep for a period of time. The twenty-year veteran said that he had been working his fourth consecutive overnight shift from ten o'clock p.m. to six o'clock a.m.[118]

Things can get very difficult when air traffic control is not functioning as it should. From a bystander's point of view, everything may seem to be operating OK. There is the normal hustle and bustle. But problems at the communication center can endanger the entire system.

Difficulties can also occur when our own personal control tower, the brain, is hampered in some way. The quality of our life mostly boils down to how well our brain can perform its duties. Scientists have now come to understand that nutrition is a major player in that process.

Most people realize that what we eat can dramatically affect our heart, liver, stomach, intestines, pancreas, arteries, etc. What is not so widely known is that food has a powerful influence on us *mentally* as well. Our moods, attitudes, emotions, and thinking ability are all affected by what we choose to place in our mouths each day.[119]

Let's look at two eaters, John and Mary. They are both thirty-five years old and lead busy lives. They make very different food choices, however, resulting in very different impacts on their brains.

> *Our moods, attitudes, emotions, and thinking ability are all affected by what we choose to place in our mouths each day.*

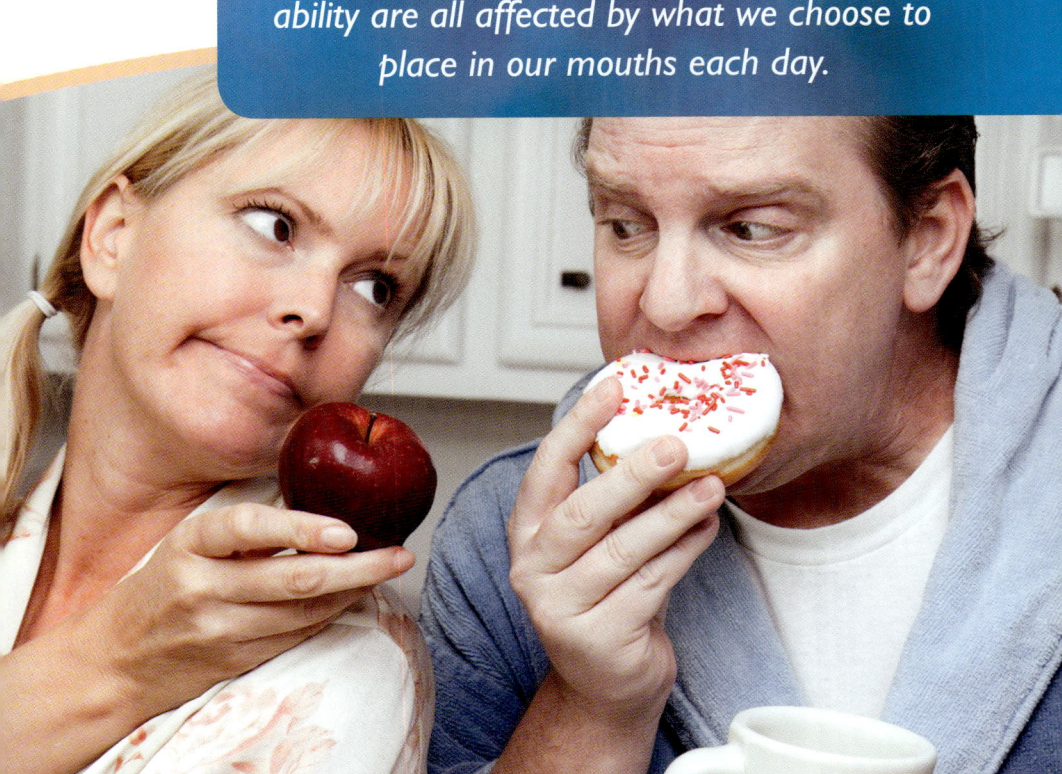

JOHN'S MEALS

John wakes up at six thirty a.m. and hurries to get ready for work. His breakfast consists of a cup of black coffee and a couple of jelly donuts from the local convenience store. For lunch, he grabs a burger and fries from a fast food restaurant with a large soda to wash it down. For supper he cooks up a steak and microwaves a frozen mac n' cheese. As a capstone to the day, he eats liberally from a bag of potato chips while watching a football game on TV.

Because this type of eating is John's regular pattern, he is elevating his risk of heart disease and other chronic ailments. But he is also putting his brain at a significant disadvantage in terms of how well he is able to cope with the demands of his workday.

The large amount of sugar in John's breakfast will give him a surge of energy and mental alertness early on but then let him down big time by midmorning, right during his crucial presentation to a new client. He could also have a hard time concentrating and assimilating new information during the late-morning staff meeting when engineers explain the new company software.[120]

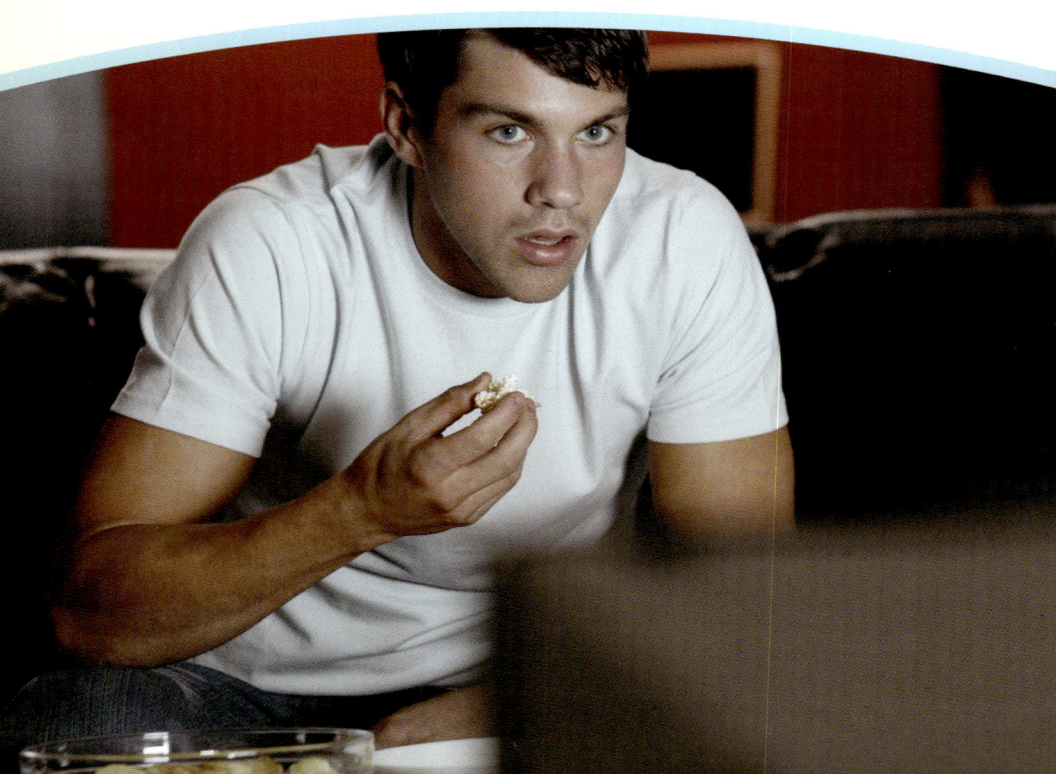

John is not doing his brain any favors by eating such a heavy dose of saturated fat for lunch and during the evening hours. Dr. Francine Grodstein, associate professor of medicine at Harvard Medical School, comments on the effects of saturated fats, "We know that's bad for your heart. There is now a lot of evidence that it is also bad for your brain."[121]

The excessive intake of harmful fats can make John more vulnerable to depression. A large European study followed the diet of more than twelve thousand people over a six-year period who had no history of depression. The participants who consumed more fast food had a 48 percent increase in their risk of depression compared with those who did not eat harmful fats.[122] Because of his choice of foods, John may have a hard time staying motivated.

Unfortunately, the damaging fats in John's diet can also adversely affect his ability to think through issues and remember details. Researchers from Brigham and Women's Hospital published a study in the journal *Annals of Neurology* where women who ate the most saturated fats from red meat and butter performed worse on tests of thinking and memory than women who ate the lowest amounts.[123]

The fat load could also make it hard for John to keep his cool when his boss criticizes him for arriving late for work five days in a row.[124]

Besides all of these problems, John has left his brain overly vulnerable to the damaging effects of what are known as "free radicals." These are the true thugs of the cranial world. Our brain typically makes up only 3 percent of our body weight but uses 20 percent of the blood supply and 25 percent of the oxygen.[125] Oxygen is used to convert the food we eat into energy. During the conversion process, some rogue oxygen molecules are released that are toxic to brain cells. They act like out-of-control bumper cars smashing into cells left and right, leaving behind a trail of wreckage.[126]

A healthy diet supplies an army of defenders against these amoral radicals, but John's food choices are providing far fewer of these vital defenders than he could have had. While he goes about his day, his brain is slowly, inexorably undergoing many more tiny assaults than necessary which, over the course of years, could ultimately lead to serious erosion of his mental capacity.[127]

CREATION HEALTH | LIFE GUIDE #8

MARY'S MEALS

Mary awakens at six o'clock a.m. from a restful sleep. After her thirty-minute exercise routine, she prepares for work, then sits down to a leisurely breakfast. The centerpiece is a cereal bowl of rolled oats that cooked in five to ten minutes. She chose it because the only ingredient on the label is "*100% Whole Grain* Rolled Oats." Mary adds almond milk [a nutritious milk substitute] and tops it with raisins and blueberries. A slice of whole wheat toast is spread with raspberry jam. She drinks a small fruit smoothie made from bananas and strawberries that are in season.

Midmorning, Mary grabs a handful of walnuts.

For lunch, she heads down to a local restaurant and orders a salad that includes spinach, cranberries, flaxseed, avocado, radishes, and cucumbers with a dressing made from extra-virgin olive oil and lemon juice. She also eats a bean/rice/tomato burrito. Water is her preferred drink.

Her afternoon snack is sunflower seeds and a crisp apple.

Supper – on the light side – consists of some lentil loaf[128] plus a small pasta salad made with shell pasta, red peppers, and broccoli. She also eats a small roll with water to drink.

Mary relaxes in the evening by eating a piece of dark chocolate and reading a best seller.

Her eating regimen revolves around fruits, vegetables, whole grains, and beans. What is going to benefit her brain the most is the *variety* of these fiber-rich foods she eats. She selects portions for each meal that are appropriate for her. The goal is not perfection, but the more consistently Mary follows this pattern, the more mental benefits she will receive. The sum is more than the individual parts.

It is also important that, unlike John who opted out of breakfast, Mary regularly eats three meals each day. A University of Bristol study revealed that individuals who ate regular meals had the best moods, worked more efficiently, and felt calmer than those who ate erratically or skipped meals.[129]

What Mary ate for breakfast got her off to a great start. Compelling evidence shows that a hearty breakfast boosts learning, memory, and psychological well-being.[130] In her book, *Eat Your Way to Happiness*, author Elizabeth Somer, MA, RD, writes, "What you choose to eat or not eat for breakfast is affecting your ability to concentrate, analyze, remember, focus and even enjoy the moment."[131]

Mary's fiber-rich morning meal will release its energy over several hours and keep her physically and mentally alert throughout the morning. She will be able to focus intently on the accounting report she has to prepare that analyzes the company's travel expenses for the last six months. She also will be able to remain calm when an angry salesperson from the field calls to report a mistake on his reimbursement for the seminar he took last month.

> *Individuals who ate regular meals had the best moods, worked more efficiently, and felt calmer than those who ate erratically or skipped meals.*

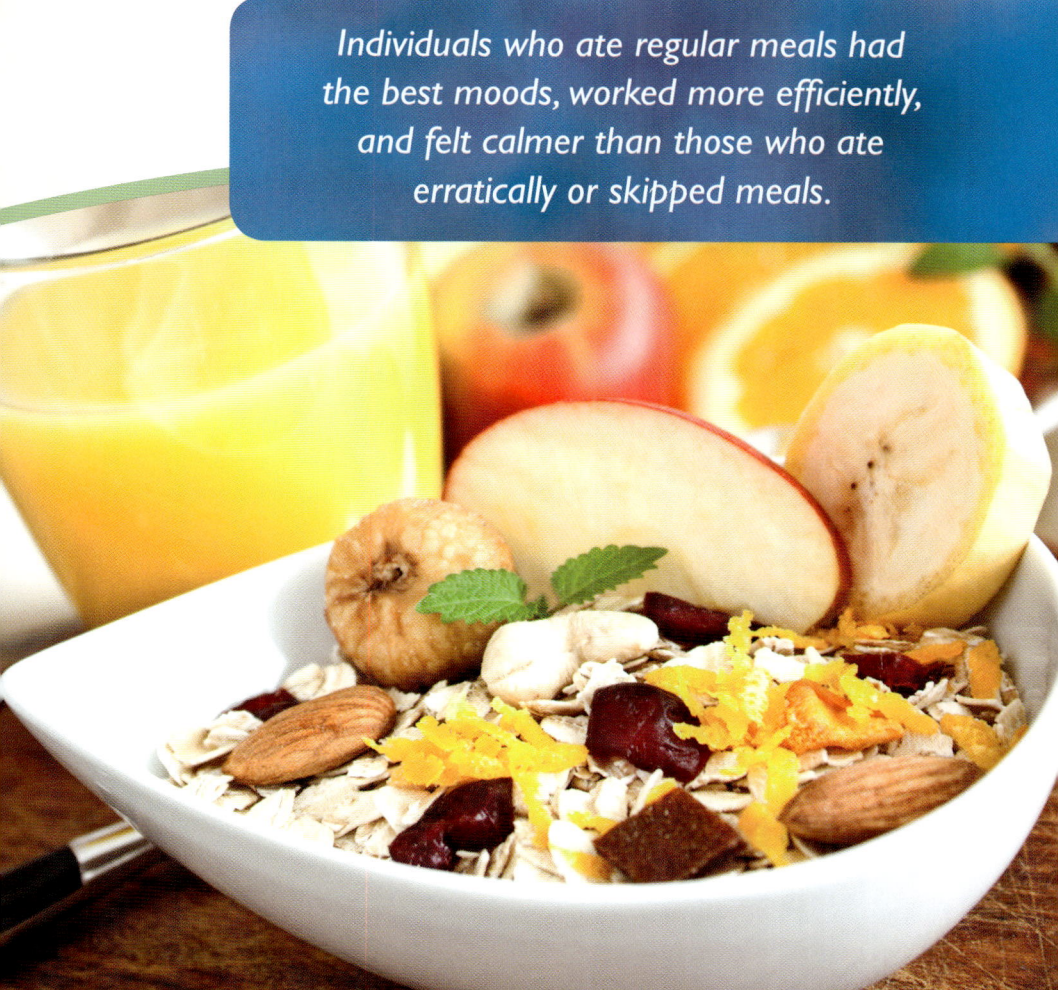

At midday, Mary's food choices for lunch of greens, berries, seeds, and vegetables plus a tasty burrito will help her maintain a positive mood and ward off depression. Diane M. Becker, director of the Center for Health Promotion at the Johns Hopkins School of Medicine, observes, "Eating a heart healthy diet – high in fiber and low in saturated fat – is a great place to start to boost your mood. There isn't any question about it." Her supper choices will help maintain that positive outlook as well.

Mary's diet is loaded with antioxidants that help her brain defend itself against the bumper-car-like free radicals that can cause so much internal damage to brain neurons and hasten memory loss and decline. The human body does not store antioxidants, but Mary's eating habits will thankfully replenish them on a regular basis.

Author Jean Carper writes, "Nature provided an army of antioxidants in the food supply. Fruits and vegetables are full of antioxidants, including vitamins and other more exotic chemicals called carotenoid and polyphenols."[132]

Mary is also benefiting from drinking water regularly. Even mild dehydration can reduce alertness, the ability to concentrate, and cognitive function.[133] Taking in water throughout the day helps her to stay focused and attentive during the typical afternoon slump.

The piece of dark chocolate that is the capstone to the day is adding to Mary's collection of "stay sharp" foods. Amy Jamieson-Petonic, RD, at Cleveland Clinic observes, "Dark chocolate is high in flavonols, a type of antioxidant that improves the blood supply to the brain and enhances cognitive skills."[134]

Most people fall somewhere in between John and Mary in their eating patterns. Wherever you find yourself on that span, the goal is to take small steps over time further away from John's type of meals and more toward Mary's. Each step on that important journey is a precious gift you give to yourself and to your amazing brain.

The apostle wrote, "Do not conform to the pattern of this world, but be transformed by the *renewing of your mind*. Then you will be able to test and approve what God's will is – his good, pleasing and perfect will" (Romans 12:2, NIV emphasis added). Usually people only apply this verse to renewing our minds spiritually. But good food plays a vital role as well. Feeding our brains with healthy foods will help us tune in to God's agenda and live out all the fullness He intended.

NOTES:

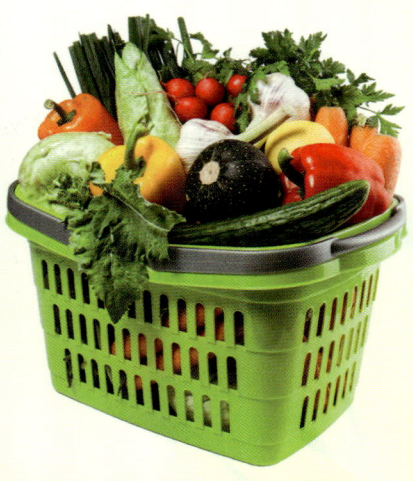

Antioxidants help the brain defend itself against free radicals that can cause so much internal damage to brain neurons and hasten memory loss and decline. Fruits and vegetables are full of antioxidants.

DISCUSSION

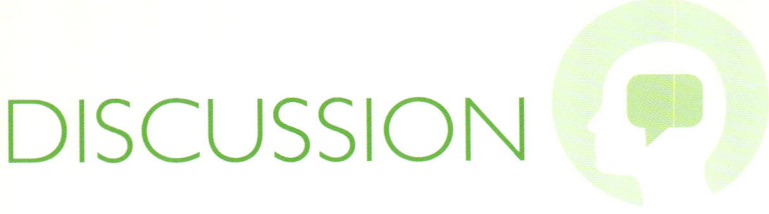

Make a list of the major differences between John and Mary's eating habits.
....
....

What caught your attention the most about how food affects us mentally? Why do you think that made an impression on you?
....
....

What connection have you noticed in your own life between what you eat and your alertness and/or mood?
....
....

In the group's own words, what are "free radicals" and why are they bad for us? What are some foods that counteract their influence?
....
....

What are some ways to help convince John to eat more healthfully? What approaches probably won't work?
....
....

What one thing from Mary's diet would be the most likely for John to incorporate besides chocolate?
....
....

How much junk food is it OK for Mary to eat?
....
....

What one thing can you do this next week to help feed your brain more healthy food?
....
....

SHARING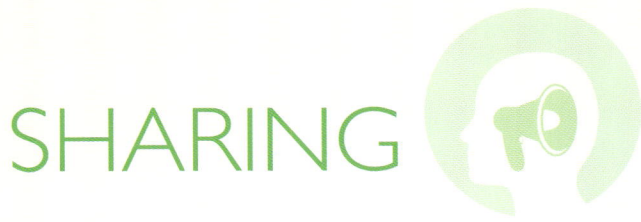

OPPORTUNITY #7:

- Pray for God to open the way for you to share something from these lessons to help someone else this week.
- Keep your radar up each day for opportunities.

ABUNDANT LIVING THOUGHT

Our moods, attitudes, emotions, and thinking ability are all affected by what we choose to place in our mouths each day.

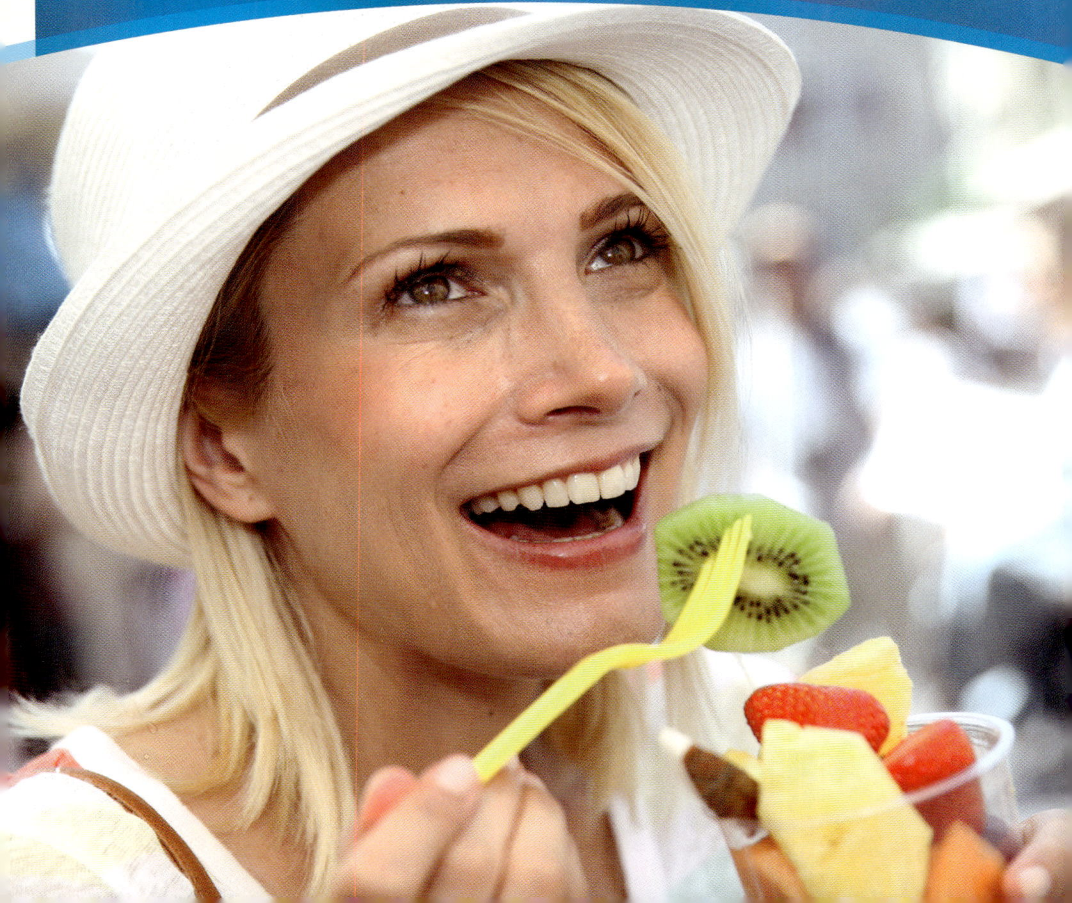

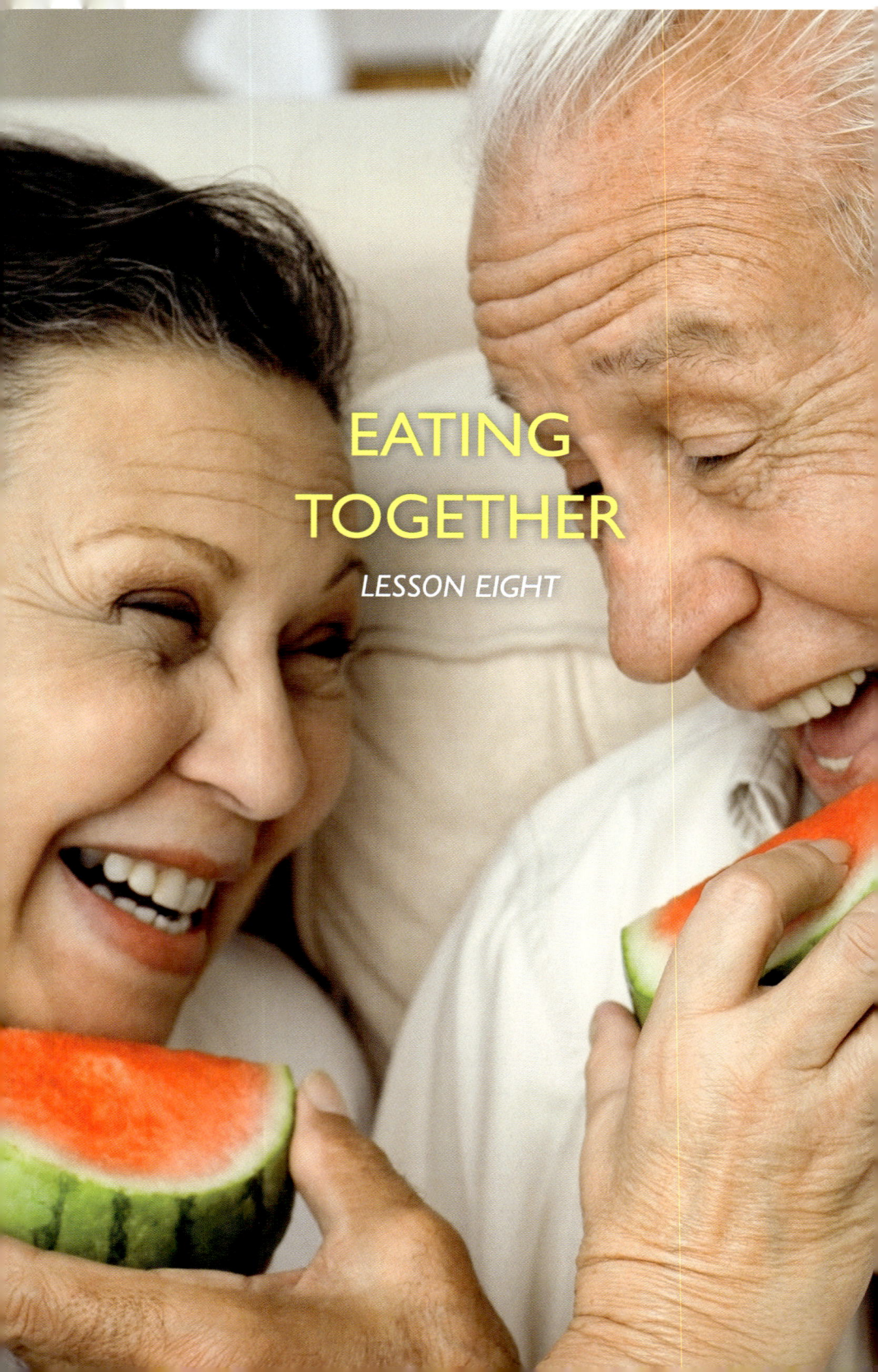
EATING TOGETHER

LESSON EIGHT

WARM UP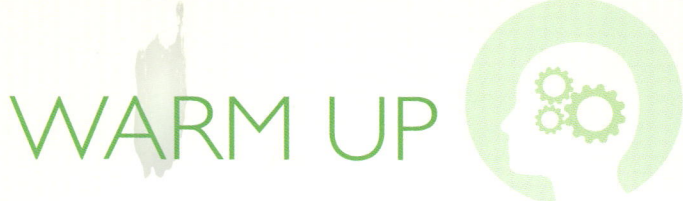

Feedback: In what ways did God open the door last week for you share some part of the lessons with someone else?

....
....
....
....

Choose one or both questions to discuss (if in group setting) or write out your answers on a separate sheet (for individual use):

1. **Share one of your most memorable moments as a member of this group.**

....
....
....

2. **What is one of the biggest benefits you have received from these lessons? Why is that meaningful for you?**

....
....
....

> *"When you eat together with family, you feast on love and laughter."*
>
> **DES CUMMINGS JR., PhD**

CREATION HEALTH | LIFE GUIDE #8

DISCOVERY

After my father's funeral, it fell to my siblings and me to sift through decades of accumulated possessions throughout my parents' home. Mom had passed away ten years earlier. We had to go through closets, dressers, chests, bags, boxes, cabinets, bundles, shelves. Everything had to be carefully perused and sorted. By the end of day one, we were all exhausted.

The next day I pulled aside the clothes in Dad's closet and spotted a series of small, worn, light-brown boxes tucked away in the back corner of the top shelf. They turned out to be a family treasure – fifteen rolls of film taken with my uncle Al's Super-8 camera forty years before during the 1950s and '60s. Too old to use with a projector, I found a place that would transfer them onto a DVD.

When the job was completed, I picked up the precious DVD and hurried home. I placed the mystery disk in our player, hit "Play," and my wife and I watched expectantly to see what, if any, images might show up on the TV. Suddenly the past came alive again, beginning with my uncle Peter's annual cookout. Long absent faces paraded across the screen in random order, hamming it up for posterity.

Without transition, the next roll started and the scene shifted. I could hardly believe my eyes. It was a Thanksgiving meal at the large dining room table in the house where I grew up. The camera slowly panned to my father, mother, sister, brother, myself, and a family from China who were very close friends. All were seated in front of a variety of dishes loaded with holiday food.

Our family had gathered around that sturdy oak table so often for shared meals, not only on special occasions but also for suppers on a regular basis. Over the years, there had been so many conversations, both silly and serious, meaningful and meaningless. So much laughter, kidding, storytelling, reporting, advice giving, speculation, squabbling, brainstorming, problem solving, sadness, and joy. The hundreds of nights we ate there are woven into the very fabric of who I am. To a large extent, we became family around that table. Those experiences helped define and anchor us. They drew us together in ways that were not fully apparent nor fully appreciated at the time.

My wife and I endeavored to carry on the tradition of eating supper together as we raised our own family. It was not without its challenges and sometimes felt like hit and miss, but it was certainly worth the effort.

Earlier in the twentieth century, it was largely taken for granted that families would gather together in the evening to eat around a common table and share conversation. However, that long-standing tradition has been seriously eroded in modern times. That mainstay of family life has been encroached upon by a variety of forces. More and more people are opting for simply placing food on a counter, then letting everyone come, fill a plate, and scatter. Or they simply eat on the run to myriad appointments.

Statistics indicate that less than one third of American families eat together more than two times per week.[135] One large study from the University of Michigan reported a 33 percent drop in family dinners from 1981 to 1997, as well as a dramatic reduction in family conversations. Among other factors redirecting children's time and attention was involvement in structured sports, which doubled the reduction, plus the time spent by children on the sidelines simply watching their siblings play, which reduced family dinners fivefold.[136]

> *So much laughter, kidding, storytelling, reporting, advice giving, speculation, squabbling, brainstorming, problem solving, sadness, and joy.*

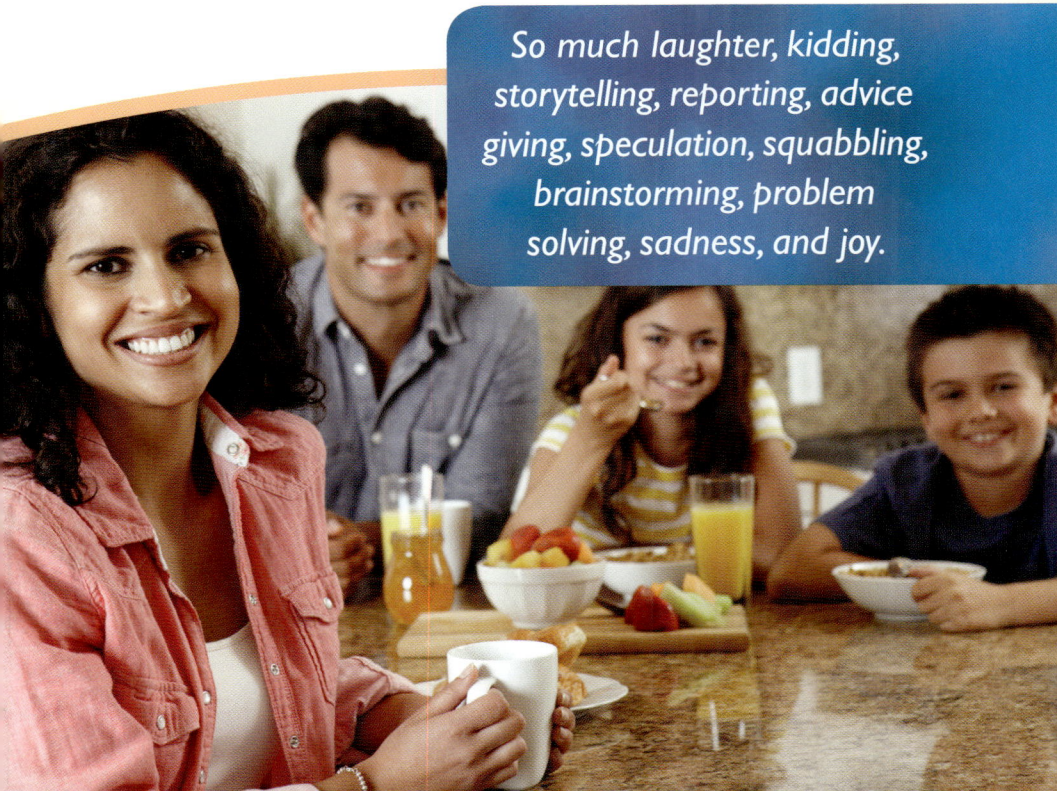

The erosion of family dinner is especially worrisome because of all the vital benefits that are being relinquished in the process. Researchers have discovered a cornucopia of good things that can happen as a result of having meals together. Such beneficial effects are all out of proportion to the seeming simplicity of the event itself. This lesson will explore several of these rather stunning findings. Hopefully, it will help those who already have dinnertime together to go deeper and will inspire those who skip it to value it sufficiently to begin with.

Dr. William Doherty, family therapist and author of numerous books on family life, observes, "The big picture is that family meals, and especially dinner, are the single most important activity that parents can do to enhance the life of their children."[137] Author and media producer Laurie David states, "Basically, everything a parent worries about can be improved by the simple act of sitting down and sharing a meal."[138]

A whole host of scientific studies confirm that kids who regularly eat family meals do much better in a surprising variety of areas. We can highlight only a few here.

The National Institutes of Health reports that a study of 99,462 sixth- to twelfth-grade students indicates that the greater the number of family meals children participate in, the lower the incidents of substance abuse, sexual activity, depression, suicide, violence, and eating disorders.[139] A study in the journal *Pediatrics* says that preschoolers' risk of obesity could be lowered by nearly 40 percent if they ate more family meals, watched less TV, and got more sleep.[140]

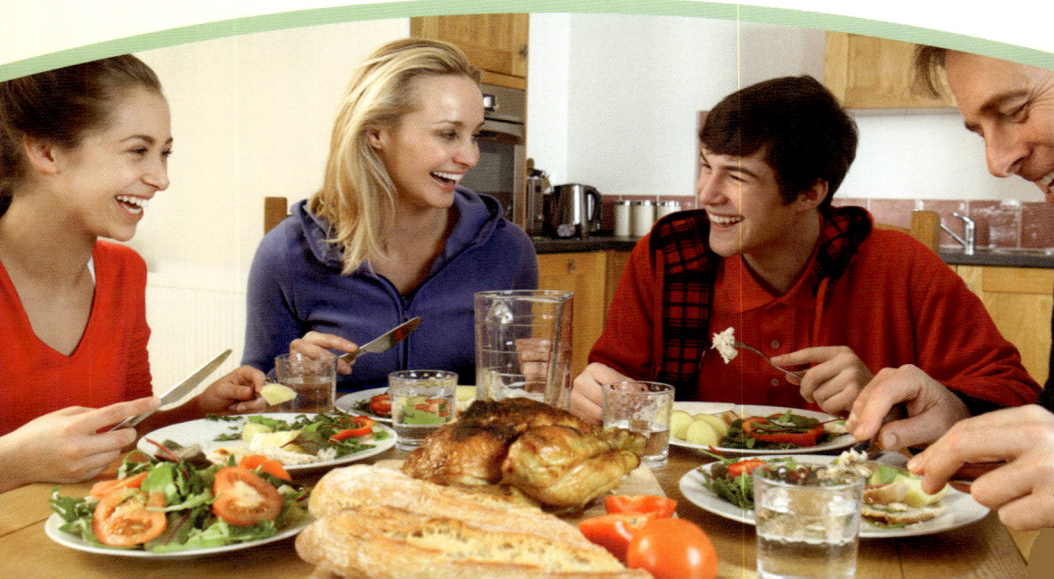

The Purdue University Center for Families reports that family meals are positively associated with higher grades, improved social skills, and greater family unity.[141] Researcher Sandra Hofferth states that the strongest predictor of academic achievement scores and low rates of behavioral problems is the frequency of family meals. It is a more important predictor than time spent in school, church, or sports.[142]

A study at Emory University showed that children who knew a lot about their family history through shared meals and other interactions had closer relationships with family members, higher self-esteem, and a greater sense of self-control.[143] Young people also build an essential sense of family identity and togetherness that enables them to feel safe and secure in an often confusing and stressful world.[144]

A year 2000 survey revealed that the more frequently nine to fourteen-year-olds had dinner with their families, the more fruits and vegetables they ate and the less soda and fried foods they consumed. Lead researcher Matthew W. Gillman, MD and director of the Obesity Prevention Program at the Harvard Medical School, says that family meals provide a great opportunity for discussion of nutrition.[145] Kids learn good food choices.

In the 1980s, the Harvard Graduate School of Education conducted a study of low-income families who had three-year-old children. They were interested in factors that influenced the size of a child's vocabulary. To their surprise, they discovered that supper was the place where children built their database of words best, even more than someone reading to them.[146]

So what can be done to make evening meals more effective or to get them started in the first place? *The following are some guidelines that people have found beneficial.* You will need to pick and choose what works best for your own particular situation. This is also an opportunity to develop your own creative approaches to what can be a challenging endeavor amid hectic, demanding schedules. If you are single, retired, or have no children, you can still benefit from the principles behind the guidelines by applying them to eating with your friends or spouse.

Make family meals a priority. It will not work for us to say we'll have family meals when we have time. They need to be written on our calendars up front with other things being planned around them as much as possible.

Sharing food together takes on special significance for Christians. After Christ's ascension, His followers are described as meeting often to eat at the same table: "Every day they continued to meet together in the temple courts. They broke bread in their homes and ate together with glad and sincere hearts" (Acts 2:46, NIV). Being delivered from this sinful world is described as participating in a grand, cosmic meal: "Blessed are those who are called to the marriage supper of the Lamb!" (Revelation 19:9, NKJV). Because of its spiritual history and symbolism, there is a sacred element to every meal. The blessings of a shared meal can apply not only to families but to any meal where people choose to partake with others.

Start small and be patient. The ideal is to have supper together five or more nights each week. But don't let that ideal keep you from doing what you can. Something is always better than nothing. We can strive toward the ideal, but any steps in the right direction are cause for cheer.

If you do not currently have a family meal tradition, begin with one meal a week or even one a month. Discuss the issue with the rest of the family and get their support. Make it fun and enjoyable. Focus at first on nights that are the least hectic.

Supper is the most impactful time because it comes at the end of the day and allows for review. But also consider putting some shared breakfasts and lunches into the mix.

Involve all family members in the process. Make it a team effort. Divide up responsibilities – choosing the food, shopping, preparation, cooking, serving, and cleanup. Alternate the responsibilities. Let the kids select the menu and do the cooking some nights all on their own. Affirm each other for trying new recipes even if they don't turn out as expected.

Make it about more than food. Simply eating at the same place at the same time is only a small part of the formula for success. It is what happens *while you eat* that counts the most. *Mealtime is more about conversation and relationships than it is about food.* Ideally, supper is the lightest meal of the day, which can allow more time to focus on interaction than on preparation.

The discussions do not need to be profound, but they do need to involve all of the people around the table in whatever direction the chatter may take, from silly to serious. Parents need to act as equals with their children at the table and enter the discussion without lecturing or admonitions. Two fun and intriguing discussion-starting resources that can help are: the "Family Dinner Box of Questions" and "Chat Pack for Kids," which are available at Amazon.com.

Model the behavior you want. Children learn values by what they observe more than what they hear. Adults can model uplifting attitudes and life-giving priorities. By their actions, adults can also informally teach conversation skills such as how to tell stories, how to listen, how to take turns speaking, how to give affirmations, and how to provide comfort and solve problems. These are skills for a lifetime.

> *Mealtime is more about conversation and relationships than it is about food.*

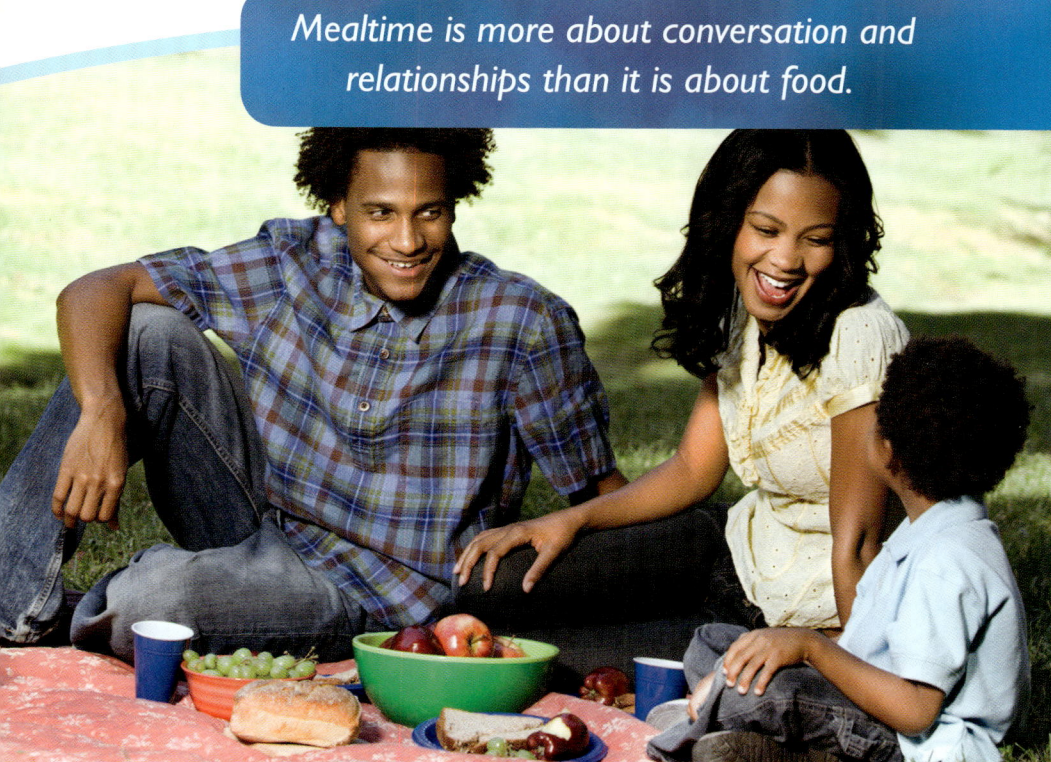

Don't force kids to eat. Nothing will turn the evening sour faster than making food a battleground. Dietitian, therapist, and author Ellyn Satter advises, "The parent is responsible for the *what, when,* and *where* of feeding, and the child is responsible for the *how much* and *whether* of eating."[147] Make sure kids are hungry enough to eat by not allowing snacks to mushroom into a substitute for the main meal.

Introduce some novelty. Mix things up such as having breakfast for supper or enjoying a picnic in the living room.

Brainstorm ideas of how to turn some meals into fun adventures. Our family still talks about the time when our daughter Stefanie was about twelve and we decided to explore French cuisine. My wife, Stef, and I were each responsible for different parts of the meal. We had to do research at the local library to be authentic. We also made a rule that we had to speak French for the first fifteen minutes. There wound up being a lot of pointing, but it was great fun.

We also had celebration dinners where we gave thanks for one of the family members without it being their birthday or a holiday. They picked their favorite foods and everyone said affirming things.

Take some time for serving others during the meal by writing encouragement cards to send out to people.

Last, turn off media. Let the TV and cell phones alone and give each other your full attention even if it is only for twenty minutes.

As children look back on their growing-up years, they won't remember the new couch we purchased or how many overtime hours we worked in order to buy them the latest gadgets. They will, however, remember the nights spent around the supper table interacting, laughing, sharing, and feeling listened to and loved.

The journey through these eight lessons on nutrition has hopefully been enlightening and instructive. Refer back to them periodically as an ongoing source of ideas to enhance your approach to eating. Make healthy choices for your own sake and for the sake of those who care about you. Small steps will become big steps over time as you continue on the path to greater fulfillment and vitality.

NOTES:

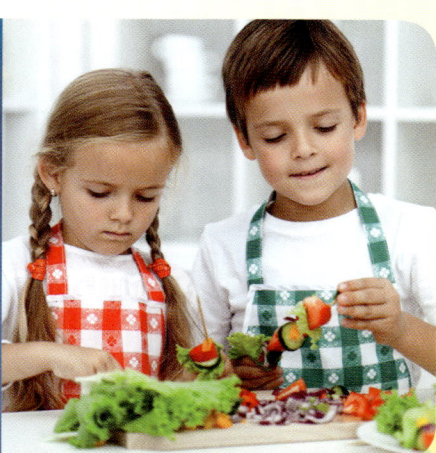

Make cooking a team effort. Let the kids select the menu and do the cooking some nights all on their own.

DISCUSSION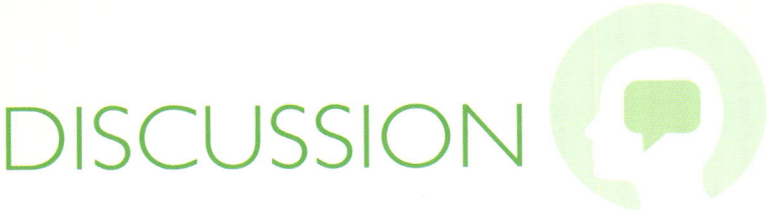

Describe one of your most positive food-related memories from your growing up years.
....
....

Share ideas of how to make family dinners a higher priority.
....
....

What are some ways to get family members to show up at the table on time and stay there?
....
....

What principles can singles or people without children get from this lesson?
....
....

What would you do if the new recipe you cooked for invited guests tasted terrible?
....
....

Describe a meal you might prepare using recipes from another country.
....
....

What would make a great shared eating experience for you?
....
....

What specific changes are you contemplating after studying these lessons?
....
....

SHARING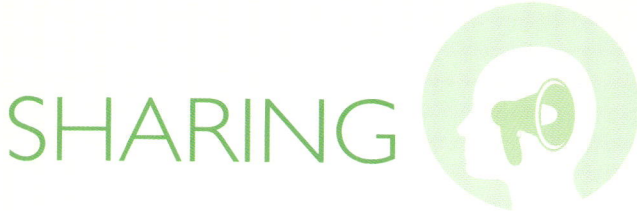

OPPORTUNITY #8:

- Pray for God to open the way for you to share something from these lessons to help someone else this week.
- Keep your radar up each day for opportunities.

ABUNDANT LIVING THOUGHT

Researchers have discovered a cornucopia of good things that can happen as a result of having meals together.

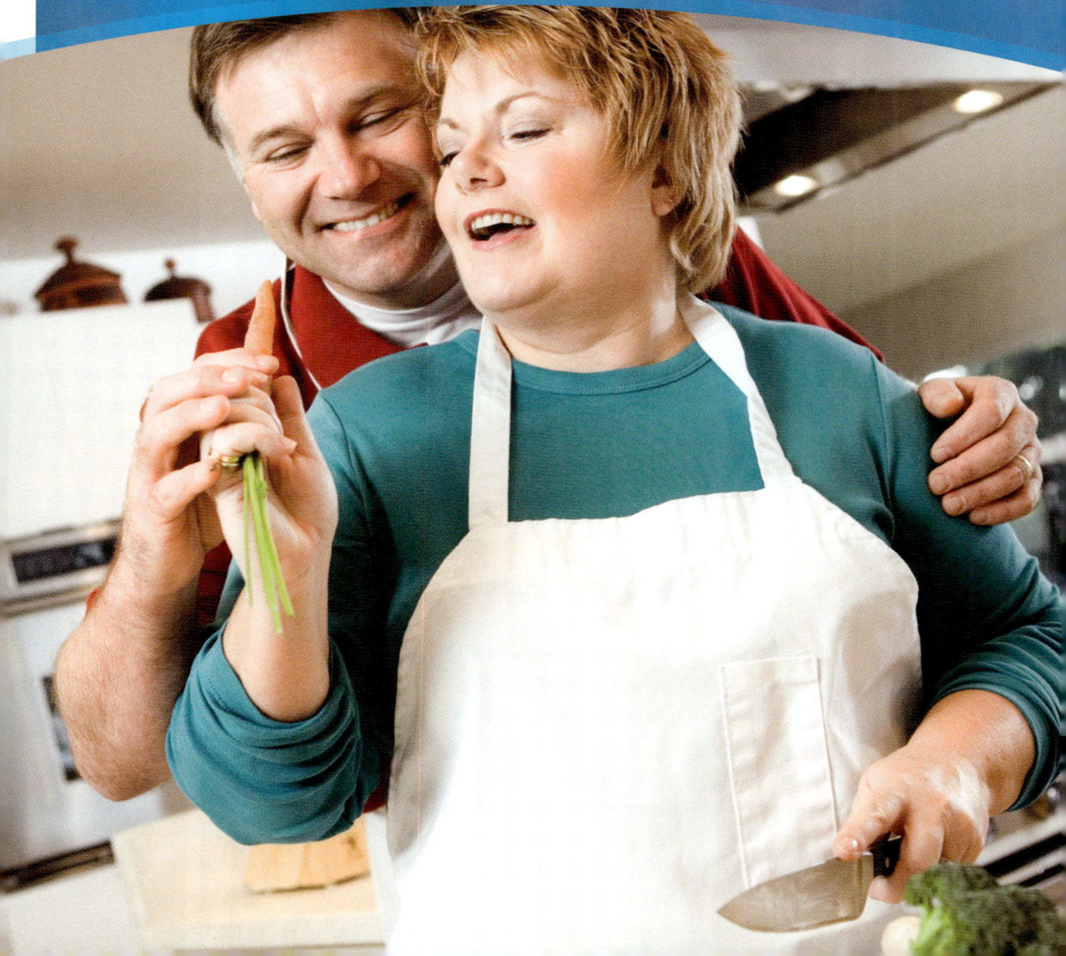

NOTES:

ABOUT THE AUTHOR

Kim Johnson is a popular writer, speaker, and fervent advocate for holistic living. As the author of three books, eleven lesson series, and many articles, his writings focus on healthy living and spiritual connectedness. His materials have been used in hundreds of churches throughout North America and internationally as well.

Johnson is an ordained minister with more than 35 years of experience as a parish pastor and church administrator. Over the years, his work with parishioners emphasized principles of whole-person health as a path to optimum mental, physical, social, and spiritual well-being. His later work with pastors and church leaders emphasized skill development such as vision casting, goal setting, support systems, relationship management, and accountability. Johnson has put his experience of working with pastors and parishioners to use in the CREATION Health Life Guide Series by creating a resource ideally suited for use in churches, small groups, or individual study.

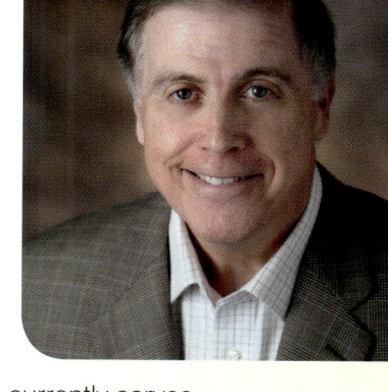

Johnson holds a Master of Divinity degree and received his Bachelor of Arts in theology. He currently serves as Director of Resource Development for churches in the state of Florida. His personal interests include reading, classical music, art and book festivals, kayaking, traveling, volunteering, and small group study. He and his wife Ann make their home in Orlando.

Author Acknowledgements: It has been a great privilege for me to be associated with the team of dedicated individuals who helped in various ways to make these CREATION Health Life Guides available. I would like to single out my wife Ann and daughter Stefanie, whose feedback and suggestions were always characterized by unfailing support and clear-eyed honesty. I have also received invaluable guidance and encouragement from Mike Cauley, Tim Nichols, Nick Howard, and Jim Epperson. Finally, I want to thank the group of local pastors who met with me personally and provided a wonderful forum for evaluating the lesson drafts.

NOTES

1. Cheryl Shireman, *What's Your Story?* (Lexington, KY: Cheryl Shireman, 2012), 43.
2. "Breaking 'Small Group Ice'," Q Place, accessed June 5, 2013, http://navigatorsdetroit.com/Ice_Breaker_Questions.pdf .
3. "How many cells are in the human body?" Dept. of Physics, University of Illinois at Urbana-Champaign, accessed June 5, 2013, http://van.physics.illinois.edu/qa/listing.php?id=17726; Elaine N. Marieb, RN, PhD, Jon Mallatt, PhD, Patricia Brady Wilhelm, PhD, *Human Anatomy* (New York, NY: Pearson Education, Inc., 2008), 26.
4. "How Big is a Trillion," LTP, accessed June 5, 2013, http://www.grc.nasa.gov/WWW/K-12/Numbers/Math/Mathematical_Thinking/how_big_is_a_trillion.htm; "Visualizing a Trillion: Just How Big That Number Is?" Digital Inspiration, accessed June 5, 2013, http://www.labnol.org/internet/visualize-numbers-how-big-is-trillion-dollars/7814/.
5. "How much is a trillion dollars?" IHTD, accessed June 5, 2013, http://ihtd.org/festivalguide/resources/how-much-is-a-trillion-dollars/.
6. "Millions, Billions, and Trillions," Courtney Taylor, About.com, accessed June 5, 2013, http://statistics.about.com/od/Applications/a/Millions-Billions-And-Trillions.htm.
7. "Blood Vessels," The Franklin Institute, accessed June 5, 2013, http://www.fi.edu/learn/heart/vessels/vessels.html; "Blood Vessels: Your Internal Superhighway," University of Rochester Medical Center, June 5, 2013, "http://www.urmc.rochester.edu/encyclopedia/content.aspx?ContentTypeID=1&ContentID=239.
8. "Treating the Troubled Heart," Vanderbilt Medicine, accessed June 5, 2013, http://www.mc.vanderbilt.edu/vanderbiltmedicine/vumc_summer05/feature1.htm.
9. "Chapter 4: Blood Vessels and Aging: The Rest of the Journey," National Institutes of Health, National Institute on Aging, accessed June 5, 2013, http://www.nia.nih.gov/health/publication/aging-hearts-and-arteries-scientific-quest/chapter-4-blood-vessels-and-aging-rest.
10. "Helping Santa Claus Get Fit," Pamela Peeke, MD, MPH, FACP, December 18, 2009, http://blogs.webmd.com/pamela-peeke-md/2009/12/helping-santa-claus-get-fit.html; "10 More Amazing Things About Our Bodies," Mercola.com, September 19, 2012, http://articles.mercola.com/sites/articles/archive/2012/09/19/10-amazing-human-body-facts.aspx.
11. "20 Most Frequently Asked Questions," The University of Utah, Genetic Science Learning Center, accessed June 5, 2013, http://learn.genetics.utah.edu/content/labs/extraction/howto/faq.html; "Amazing Human Facts," HubPages, accessed June 5, 2013, http://vinodpaulson.hubpages.com/hub/AMAZING_HUMAN_FACTS.
12. "DNA," Biology Reference.com, June 5, 2013, http://www.biologyreference.com/Co-Dn/DNA.html.
13. "How Genes Work," National Institute of General Medical Sciences, NIH, accessed June 5, 2013, http://publications.nigms.nih.gov/thenewgenetics/chapter1.html.
14. "100 Trillion Connections: New Efforts Probe and Map the Brain's Detailed Architecture," Carl Zimmer, *Scientific American*, accessed June 5, 2013, http://www.scientificamerican.com/article.cfm?id=100-trillion-connections; "Children and Brain Development: What We Know How Children Learn," Judith Graham, The University of Maine, Cooperative Extension Publications, accessed June 5, 2013, http://umaine.edu/publications/4356e/.

15. "New imaging method developed at Stanford reveals stunning details of brain connections," Bruce Goldman, Stanford School of Medicine, November 17, 2010, http://med.stanford.edu/ism/2010/november/neuron-imaging.html.
16. "Lungs," National Geographic, accessed June 5, 2013, http://science.nationalgeographic.com/science/health-and-human-body/human-body/lungs-article/; "Your Lungs and Respiratory System," KidsHealth, accessed June 5, 2013, http://kidshealth.org/kid/htbw/lungs.html#.
17. Jason James Taylor, BSc, MSc, Barbara Janson Cohen, BA, MSEd, *Structure and Function of the Human Body, 10th Edition* (New York, NY: Lippincott Williams & Wilkins, 2013), 345.
18. Susan E. Mulroney, PhD, Adam K. Myers, PhD, *Essential Physiology* (Philadelphia, PA: Saunders Elsevier, 2009), 274.
19. Ibid., 279.
20. "Your Digestive System and How It Works," US Department of Health and Human Services, accessed June 5, 2013, http://digestive.niddk.nih.gov/ddiseases/pubs/yrdd/.
21. Taylor & Cohen, *Structure and Function*, 344.
22. Elaine N. Marieb, RN, PhD, Jon Mallatt, PhD, Patricia Brady Wilhelm, PhD, *Human Anatomy*, 647, 668.
23. "Healthy Gut Bacteria," Science Learning, accessed June 5, 2013, http://www.sciencelearn.org.nz/Contexts/Digestion-Chemistry/Looking-Closer/Healthy-gut-bacteria.
24. Cheryl Shireman, *What's Your Story?* (Lexington, KY: Cheryl Shireman, 2012), 52.
25. Barbara Ann Kipfer, *4,000 questions for getting to know anyone and everyone* (New York, NY: Random House Reference, 2004), 83.
26. "5 Ways to Enjoy Eating & Savor Your Food," Margarita Tartakovsky, MS, accessed June 5, 2013, PsychCentral, http://blogs.psychcentral.com/weightless/2012/07/5-ways-to-enjoy-eating-savor-your-food/.
27. "The Pleasures of Eating," Kimerer LaMothe, PhD, *Psychology Today,* May 15, 2010, http://www.psychologytoday.com/blog/what-body-knows/201005/the-pleasures-eating.
28. "Taste Science," George Herbert, Cornell University, accessed June 5, 2013, http://www.tastescience.com/BookExpoBrochure06-2.pdf .
29. "The Science Behind How We Taste," Heather Hatfield, WebMD, accessed June 5, 2013, http://www.webmd.com/diet/features/science-how-we-taste.
30. "Where Did Pentecost Come From?" Dr. Ray Pritchard, Jesus.org, accessed June 5, 2013, http://www.jesus.org/early-church-history/pentecost/where-did-pentecost-come-from.htm.
31. Mitch and Zhava Glaser, *The Fall Feasts of Israel* (Chicago, IL: Moody Publishers, 1987), 162.
32. "Instead of Eating to Diet, They're Eating to Enjoy," Tara Parker-Pope, *The New York Times*, September 16, 2008, http://www.nytimes.com/2008/09/17/dining/17diet.html?_r=2&.
33. "5 Ways to Enjoy Eating and Savor Your Food," Margarita Tartakovsky, MS, PsychCentral, accessed June 5, 2013, http://blogs.psychcentral.com/weightless/2012/07/5-ways-to-enjoy-eating-savor-your-food/.

34. "PsychCentral's Slow Eating Challenge: Are You Ready to Enjoy Food Again?" Victoria Gigante, EdM, Psych Central, accessed June 5, 2013, http://psychcentral.com/blog/archives/2012/05/03/psychcentrals-slow-eating-challenge-are-you-ready-to-enjoy-food-again/; "Does the number of times I chew my food impact my digestion?" World's Healthiest Foods,com, accessed June 5, 2013, http://www.whfoods.com/genpage.php?tname=george&dbid=36 .

35. "Savoring Food – Eating for Enjoyment and Satisfaction," Kathy Nichols, Ezine Articles, accessed June 5, 2013, http://ezinearticles.com/?Savoring-Food---Eating-for-Enjoyment-and-Satisfaction&id=1070798.

36. "Color Your Plate with Blueberries," Ivonne Cueva, Academy of Nutrition and Dietetics, accessed June 5, 2013, http://www.eatright.org/nnm/blog.aspx?id=4294970053&blogid=6442450952&terms=blueberries; "Blueberries and Health," Peggy Trowbridge Filippone, About.com, accessed June 5, 2013, http://homecooking.about.com/od/foodhealthinformation/a/blueberryhealth.htm; "History and Facts of Blueberries," Rhonda Cassaday, April 2, 2009, http://business.intuit.com/directory/article-history-and-facts-on-blueberries.

37. Teresa Fung, ScD, RD, *Reducing Sugar and Salt* (Boston, MA: Harvard Health Publications, 2012), 25.

38. "How to Know When Your Stomach Is Full & Stop Eating," Serena Styles, San *Francisco Chronicle*, http://healthyeating.sfgate.com/stomach-full-stop-eating-3080.html.

39. "Healthy Eating: Recognizing Your Hunger Signals," http://www.mypatientpoint.com/nutrition-eating/healthy-eating-recognizing-your-hunger-signals?secId=zx3302.

40. "Savoring Food," Kathy Nichols, http://ezinearticles.com/?Savoring-Food---Eating-for-Enjoyment-and-Satisfaction&id=1070798.

41. CF "Ice Breaker Questions," accessed June 5, 2013, http://jimhough.com/cf/ibquestions.html.

42. Jennifer Carter, Over 600 *Icebreakers & Games* (Lexington, KY: Jennifer Carter, 2012), 67.

43. Pioppi, "Italy Tourism," accessed June 5, 2013, http://www.cilento-travel.com/en/cilento/charming-resorts/pioppi.html.

44. "The Mediterranean Diet," Kathleen M. Zelman, MPH, RD, LD, WebMD, accessed June 5, 2013, http://www.webmd.com/food-recipes/guide/the-mediterranean-diet.

45. "Nutrition News: Mediterraneans abandon their famous diet," Harvard School of Public Health, accessed June 5, 2013, http://www.hsph.harvard.edu/news/hsph-in-the-news/mediterraneans-abandon-diet-willett/.

46. "Mediterraneans Abandon Their Famous Diet," Jeremy Cherfas, July 14, 2011, http://www.npr.org/2011/07/14/137823222/mediterraneans-abandon-their-famous-diet.

47. "Nutrition News," HSPH, http://www.hsph.harvard.edu/news/hsph-in-the-news/mediterraneans-abandon-diet-willett/.

48. "Overweight and Obesity," Centers for Disease Control and Prevention, accessed June 5, 2013, http://www.cdc.gov/obesity/data/childhood.html.

49. Gene Stone, *Forks Over Knives* (New York, NY: The Experiment, 2011), 4; "National Diabetes Fact Sheet, 2011," Centers for Disease Control, http://www.cdc.gov/diabetes/pubs/pdf/ndfs_2011.pdf .

50. Gene Stone, *Forks Over Knives*, 17.

51. "Healthy Eating," American Diabetes Association, accessed June 5, 2013, http://www.diabetes.org/diabetes-basics/prevention/checkup-america/healthy-eating.html.
52. "Eating Well and Losing Weight," American Heart Association, accessed June 5, 2013, http://www.heart.org/HEARTORG/Conditions/More/CardiacRehab/Eating-Well-and-Losing-Weight_UCM_307096_Article.jsp.
53. "Quiz: How Healthy is Your Diet?" American Institute for Cancer Research, accessed June 5, 2013, http://www.aicr.org/reduce-your-cancer-risk/diet/reduce_diet_quiz.html.
54. Stuart A. Seale, M.D., Teresa Sherard, M.D., Diana Fleming, Ph.D., LDN, *The Full Plate Diet* (Austin, TX: Bard Press, 2010), 83.
55. "The Benefits of Fiber: For Your Heart, Weight, and Energy," Kathleen M. Zelman, MPH, RD, LD, WebMD, accessed June 5, 2013, http://www.webmd.com/diet/fiber-health-benefits-11/fiber-weight-control?page=1.
56. "Dietary Fiber: Essential for a healthy diet," Mayo Clinic, accessed June 5, 2013, http://www.mayoclinic.com/health/fiber/NU00033; "The benefits of fiber," Nancy Anderson, Emory HeartWise Program, accessed June 5, 2013, http://www.emory.edu/EMORY_REPORT/erarchive/1996/May/ERmay.6/5_6_96wellness.html; "Increasing Fiber Intake," University of California San Francisco Medical Center, accessed June 5, 2013, "http://www.ucsfhealth.org/education/increasing_fiber_intake/index.html.
57. Seale, et al., *The Full Plate Diet*, 43.
58. "Dr. Andrew Weil's 5 Holistic Health Secrets," *The Dr OZ Show*, accessed June 5, 2013, http://www.doctoroz.com/videos/dr-andrew-weil-5-holistic-health-secrets?page=2; "Dr. Andrew Weil's Diet," WebMD, accessed June 5, 2013, http://www.webmd.com/diet/dr-andrew-weil-what-it-is; "Fiber – Nature's Secret to Weight Loss," Jeff Greenberg, MD, September 13, 2012, http://drjeffgreenberg.com/tag/fiber/; Seale, et al., *The Full Plate Diet*, 24; Darlene Blaney, MSc, NCP and Hans Diehl, DrHSc, MPH, FACN, *The Optimal Diet* (Hagerstown, MD: Autumn House Publishing, 2009), 10.
59. "Fiber and Children's Diets," American Heart Association, accessed June 5, 2013, http://www.heart.org/HEARTORG/GettingHealthy/NutritionCenter/Fiber-and-Childrens-Diets_UCM_305981_Article.jsp.
60. "Increasing Fiber Intake," University of California San Francisco Medical Center, accessed June 5, 2013, http://www.ucsfhealth.org/education/increasing_fiber_intake/index.html.
61. Monica Reed, MD, *The Creation Health Breatkthrough* (New York, NY: Center Street, 2007), 192.
62. USDA National Nutrition Database for Standard Reference, Fiber, Total Directory, http://www.nal.usda.gov/fnic/foodcomp/Data/SR17/wtrank/sr17a291.pdf ; Sharon Palmer, RD, "The Top Fiber-Rich Food List," *Today's Dietitian*, July 2008, http://www.todaysdietitian.com/newarchives/063008p28.shtml; "Chart of High-Fiber Foods," Mayo Clinic, accessed June 5, 2013, http://www.mayoclinic.com/health/high-fiber-foods/NU00582.
63. Editors of Whole Living Magazine, *Powerfoods* (New York, NY: Clarkson Potter/Publishers, 2010), 20.
64. "Chart of High-Fiber Foods," Mayo Clinic, accessed June 5, 2013, http://www.mayoclinic.com/health/high-fiber-foods/NU00582; "Fiber Content of Foods in Common Portions," Harvard University Health Services, accessed June 5, 2013, http://huhs.harvard.edu/assets/file/ourservices/service_nutrition_fiber.pdf.

65. Jennifer Carter, Over 600 *Ice-Breakers & Games* (Lexington, KY, Jennifer Carter, 2012), 38.
66. Garry Poole, *The Complete Book of Questions* (Grand Rapids, MI: Zondervan, 2003), 90.
67. Barbara Rolls, PhD, *The Ultimate Volumetrics Diet* (New York, NY: William Morrow, 2012), 18–19.
68. "Water Content of Fruits and Vegetables," Sandra Bastin and Kim Henken, December, 1997, Cooperative Extension Service, University of Kentucky College of Agriculture, http://www.ca.uky.edu/enri/pubs/enri129.pdf.
69. "Energy Density and Weight Loss: Feel full on fewer calories," Mayo Clinic Staff, accessed June 5, 2013, http://www.mayoclinic.com/health/weight-loss/NU00195.
70. "Decreasing Consumption of Energy Dense Foods," Shape Up America!, accessed June 5, 2013, http://www.shapeup.org/resources/sus_energy.html.
71. Walt Larimore, MD, Sherri Flynt, MPH, RD, LD, *SuperSized Kids* (New York: NY, Center Street, 2005), 132.
72. http://www.choosemyplate.gov/.
73. Seale et al., *The Full Plate Diet*, 76–81.
74. "Eat Your Vegetables: 15 Tips for Veggie Haters," Elaine Magee, MPH, RD, WebMD, accessed June 5, 2013, http://www.webmd.com/diet/features/eat-your-vegetables-15-tips-for-veggie-haters.
75. "Basic Nutrition: High-Fiber Foods," Shereen Jegtvig, About.com, accessed June 5, 2013, http://nutrition.about.com/od/foodfun/a/high_fiber_food.htm.
76. "30 Tricks to Make Fiber Taste Better," Elizabeth Ward, Men's Health.com, accessed June 5, 2013, http://www.menshealth.com/mhlists/high_fiber_foods/index.php.
77. "Fiber: Start Roughing It," Harvard School of Public Health, accessed June 5, 2013, http://www.hsph.harvard.edu/nutritionsource/fiber-full-story/.
78. "How to Lose Weight By Eating Fruits and Vegetables," Anne Baley, eHow.com, accessed June 5, 2013, http://www.ehow.com/how_5187204_lose-weight-eating-fruits-vegetables.html.
79. "How to Start Eating Healthier," Leanne Beattie, SparkPeople.com, accessed June 5, 2013, http://www.sparkpeople.com/resource/nutrition_articles.asp?id=1011.
80. Madeleine S. Miller and J. Lane Miller, *Harper's Bible Dictionary* (New York, NY: Harper & Row, Publishers, 1961), 57; *Everyday Life in Bible Times* (Washington, DC: National Geographic Society, 1967), 273.
81. Cheryl Shireman, *What's Your Story* (Lexington, KY: Cheryl Shireman, 2012), 77.
82. Barbara Ann Kipfer, *4,000 Questions for Getting to Know Anyone and Everyone* (New York, NY: Random House Reference, 2004), 100.
83. "Eating Healthier and Feeling Better Using the Nutrition Facts Label," US FDA.gov, accessed June 5, 2013, http://www.fda.gov/Food/ResourcesForYou/Consumers/ucm266853.htm.
84. "Deciphering Food Labels," Kids Health from Nemours, accessed June 5, 2013, http://kidshealth.org/parent/nutrition_center/healthy_eating/food_labels.html#.
85. "How to Understand and Use the Nutrition Facts Label," US Food and Drug Administration, accessed June 5, 2013, http://www.fda.gov/food/ResourcesForYou/Consumers/NFLPM/ucm274593.htm.

86. "The Basics of the Nutrition Facts Panel," Academy of Nutrition and Dietetics, Eat Right, January 2013, http://www.eatright.org/public/content.aspx?id=10935 .
87. "What are MUFA's, and should I include them in my diet?" Katherine Zeratsky, RD, LD, Mayo Clinic, accessed June 5, 2013, http://www.mayoclinic.com/health/mufas/AN02120; "Fats and Cholesterol," Harvard School of Public Health: The Nutrition Source, accessed June 5, 2013, http://www.hsph.harvard.edu/nutritionsource/fats-full-story/.
88. "Shining the Spotlight on Trans Fats," Harvard School of Public Health, The Nutrition Source, accessed June 5, 2013, http://www.hsph.harvard.edu/nutritionsource/transfats/.
89. "How food manufacturers trick consumers with deceptive ingredients lists," Mike Adams, July 10, 2007, http://www.naturalnews.com/021929_groceries_food_products.html.
90. "Parent Communications – Balanced Diet Theme," HSPH, accessed June 5, 2013, http://www.hsph.harvard.edu/prc/files/2012/09/04parentresgoforwholegrain.pdf.
91. "Whole grains make a difference," USDA.gov, accessed June 5, 2013, http://www.fns.usda.gov/fns/corenutritionmessages/Files/how_to_tell_whole_grain.pdf.
92. "Dietary Fiber," Sherry Henley, Scottie Misner, University of Arizona College of Agriculture and Life Sciences, August 1999, http://cals.arizona.edu/pubs/health/az1127.html.
93. "Sugary Drinks or Diet Drinks: What's the Best Choice?" Harvard School of Public Health, accessed June 5, 2013, http://www.hsph.harvard.edu/nutritionsource/sugary-vs-diet-drinks/.
94. "Sugar Addiction," Alexis Conason, PsyD, Psychologytoday.com, "Eating Mindfully," April 4, 2012, http://www.psychologytoday.com/blog/eating-mindfully/201204/sugar-addiction.
95. "Added Sugar: What You Need To Know," American Academy of Family Physicians, Family Doctor.org, accessed June 5, 2013, http://familydoctor.org/familydoctor/en/prevention-wellness/food-nutrition/sugar-and-substitutes/added-sugar-what-you-need-to-know.html.
96. "Sugars 101," American Heart Association, accessed June 5, 2013, http://www.heart.org/HEARTORG/GettingHealthy/NutritionCenter/Sugars-101_UCM_306024_Article.jsp; Kimberly Lord Stewart, *Eating Between the Lines* (New York, NY: St. Martins Press, 2007), 269.
97. "What Eating Too Much Sugar Does to Your Brain," David DiSalvo, PsychologyToday.com, accessed June 5, 2013, http://www.psychologytoday.com/collections/201207/food-thought/how-sugar-hurts-the-brain.
98. Teresa Fung, ScD, RD, *Reducing Sugar and Salt* (Boston, MA: Harvard Health Publications, 2012), 25.
99. "How to Spot Added Sugar On Food Labels," Harvard School of Public Health, accessed June 5, 2013, http://www.hsph.harvard.edu/nutritionsource/added-sugar-on-food-labels/ ; United State Department of Agriculture, "Dietary Guidelines for Americans 2005," Chapter 7 Carbohydrates, accessed June 5, 2013, http://www.health.gov/DietaryGuidelines/dga2005/document/html/chapter7.htm.
100. "Processed Foods: Where is all that salt coming from?" American Heart Association, February 23, 2012, http://www.heart.org/HEARTORG/Conditions/HighBloodPressure/PreventionTreatmentofHighBloodPresssure/Processed-Foods-Where-is-all-that-salt-coming-from_UCM_426950_Article.jsp.

101. Kimberly Lord Stewart, *Eating Between the Lines* (New York, NY: St. Martins Press, 2007), 223.
102. CF "Ice Breaker" Questions, http://jimhough.com/cf/ibquestions.html.
103. "Ice Breaker and Group Openers," Fair Haven LifeGroups, accessed June 5, 2013, http://www.fhmin.org/clientimages/48137/ice%20breakers%20and%20group%20openers.pdf.
104. "9 Tips to Save Money on your Grocery Bill," Nicole Cherie Jones, accessed June 5, 2013, http://www.rachaelraymag.com/food-how-to/grocery-shopping-tips/9-tips-to-save-money-on-your-grocery-bill.
105. "15 Ways Supermarkets Trick You Into Spending More Money," Gus Lubin, Business Insider, July 26, 2011, http://www.businessinsider.com/supermarkets-make-you-spend-money-2011-7?op=1.
106. Mary Ostyn, *Family Feasts for $75 a week* (Birmingham, AL: Oxmoor House, Inc., 2009), 8, 11.
107. Steve & Annette Economides, *Cut Your Grocery Bill In Half* (Nashville, TN: Thomas Nelson, 2010), 22.
108. "Use Grocery List to Save Time, Eat Healthier," Alice Henneman, Nebraska Nutrition Education Program, accessed June 5, 2013, http://food.unl.edu/web/fnh/grocery-list.
109. Mary Ostyn, *Family Feasts*, 38.
110. "Unit Price," UMass.edu, accessed June 5, 2013, http://www.umass.edu/nibble/infofile/unitpric.html.
111. "12 Ways to Save Money on Food Shopping," Kathleen M. Zelman, MPH, RD, LD, WebMD, accessed June 5, 2013, http://www.webmd.com/food-recipes/guide/10-ways-save-money-food-shopping.
112. Jonni McCoy, *Miserly Moms* (Minneapolis, MN: Bethany House, 2009), 97.
113. "Tips for Vegetarians," United States Department of Agriculture, ChooseMyPlate.gov, accessed June 5, 2013, http://www.choosemyplate.gov/healthy-eating-tips/tips-for-vegetarian.html.
114. Steve & Annette Economides, *Cut Your Grocery Bill In Half*, 138.
115. Feeding Your Children," Editors PureHealthMD," HowStuffWorks.com, accessed June 5, 2013, http://health.howstuffworks.com/pregnancy-and-parenting/feeding-your-children.htm.
116. Cheryl Shireman, *What's Your Story?* (Lexington, KY: Cheryl Shireman, 2012), 50.
117. Barbara Ann Kipfer, *4,000 Questions for Getting to Know Anyone and Everyone* (New York, NY: Random House Reference, 2004), 23.
118. "Air Traffic Controller Is Suspended," Timothy Williams and Jad Mouawad, NYTimes.com, March 24, 2011, http://www.nytimes.com/2011/03/25/us/25airport.html?pagewanted=all&_r=0; "NTSB: Air traffic controller fell asleep, leaving plane on their own," CNN, March 25, 2011, http://www.cnn.com/2011/TRAVEL/03/24/dc.air.traffic.suspension/index.html.
119. "Natural mood foods: The actions of polyphenols against psychiatric and cognitive disorders," Fernando Gomez-Pinilla and Trang T Nguyen, National Institutes of Health, January 7, 2012, http://www.ncbi.nlm.nih.gov/pmc/articles/PMC3355196/.
120. "A Better Breakfast Can Boost a Child's Brainpower," Allison Aubrey, September 6, 2004, script of NPR interview, http://www.npr.org/templates/story/story.php?storyId=5738848 .

121. "Boost your memory by eating right," Harvard Health Publications, August 2012, http://www.health.harvard.edu/newsletters/Harvard_Womens_Health_Watch/2012/August/boost-your-memory-by-eating-right.

122. "Nutrition and depression at the forefront of progress," TA Popa and M Ladea, US National Library of Medicine, *Journal of Medicine and Life*, December 25, 2012, http://www.ncbi.nlm.nih.gov/pmc/articles/PMC3539842/.

123. "Boost your memory by eating right," Harvard Health Publications, August 2012, http://www.health.harvard.edu/newsletters/Harvard_Womens_Health_Watch/2012/August/boost-your-memory-by-eating-right.

124. "How to Eat Smart," Randy Blaun, Andreas Wiesenack, *Psychology Today*, reviewed July 20, 2012, http://www.psychologytoday.com/collections/201207/food-thought/how-eat-smart.

125. "Exercise And The Brain," Jeffrey Kleim, PhD, March 2011, http://www.ideafit.com/fitness-library/exercise-and-the-brain.

126. "How to Eat Smart," Randy Blaun, Andreas Wiesenack, *Psychology Today*, reviewed July 20, 2012, http://www.psychologytoday.com/collections/201207/food-thought/how-eat-smart.

127. "How to Save Your Brain," Nikhil Swaminathan, January 1, 2012, *Psychology Today*, http://www.psychologytoday.com/collections/201207/food-thought/eat-save-your-brain.

128. See http://vegetarian.about.com/od/maindishentreerecipes/r/ricelentilloaf.htm, and http://www.tasteofhome.com/recipes/lentil-loaf.

129. Elizabeth Somer, MA, RD, *Eat Your Way to Happiness* (Ontario, Canada: Harlequin Enterprises Limited, 2009), 36.

130. Jean Carper, *Your Miracle Brain* (New York, NY: HarperCollins Publishers, 2000), 112.

131. Somer, *Eat Your Way to Happiness*, 47.

132. Carper, *Your Miracle Brain*, 149.

133. Bar-David Y, Urkin J. Kozminsky E, "The effect of voluntary dehydration on cognitive functions of elementary school children," *Acta Paediatr*, 2005 Nov; 94(11): 1667–73, http://www.ncbi.nlm.nih.gov/pubmed/16303708; "Dangers of Dehydration," Creation Health, accessed June 5, 2012, http://creationhealth.com/CREATIONHealth/Nutrition/DangersofDehydration/tabid/3005/Default.aspx.

134. "How can diet help your brain? Let us count the ways," Amy Jamieson-Petonic, RD, Cleveland Clinic, accessed June 5, 2012, http://my.clevelandclinic.org/giving/news-events/publications/catalyst_e_news/archive/7-2/food-for-thought.aspx.

135. Marshall P. Duke, Robyn Fivush, Amber Lazarua, and Jennifer Bohanek, "Of Ketchup and Kin: Dinnertime Conversations as a Major Source of Family Knowledge, Family Adjustment, and Family Resilience," May 2003, Department of Psychology, Emory University, http://www.marial.emory.edu/pdfs/Duke_Fivush027-03.pdf .

136. John F. Sandberg, and Sandra L. Hofferth, "Changes in Children's Time with Parents," US 1981–1997, Population Studies Center at the Institute for Social Research, University of Michigan, May 2001, http://www.psc.isr.umich.edu/pubs/pdf/rr01-475.pdf.

137. "Shared Meals, Shared Lives: The Importance of Family Dinner," Tamera Schreur, accessed June 5, 2013, http://familytherapyinwestchester.com/1/archives/02-2011/1.html.
138. "Getting Closer to Your Kids One Meal at a Time," How's Your Family.com, accessed June 5, 2013, http://howsyourfamily.com/getting-closer-to-your-kids-one-meal-at-a-time/.
139. Fulkerson JA, Story M, Mellin A, Leffert N, Neumark-Sztainer D, French SA, US National Library of Medicine, National Institutes of Health, *Journal of Adolescent Health*, September 2006, http://www.ncbi.nlm.nih.gov/pubmed/16919794?dopt=Abstact.
140. "Less TV, More Family Dinners Fight Childhood Obesity," Bill Hendrick, WebMD, accessed June 5, 2013, http://www.webmd.com/parenting/news/20100208/less-tv-more-family-dinners-fight-childhood-obesity.
141. "Promoting Family Meals," Purdue University Center for Families, accessed June 5, 2013, http://www.cfs.purdue.edu/CFF/promotingfamilymeals/index.html.
142. Marshall P. Duke, Robyn Fivush, Amber Lazarua, and Jennifer Bohanek, "Of Ketchup and Kin: Dinnertime Conversations as a Major Source of Family Knowledge, Family Adjustment, and Family Resilience," May 2003, Department of Psychology, Emory University, http://www.marial.emory.edu/pdfs/Duke_Fivush027-03.pdf.
143. "Family Nutrition: The Truth About Family Meals," Larry Forthun, University of Florida IFAS Extension, accessed June 5, 2013, http://edis.ifas.ufl.edu/pdffiles/FY/FY106100.pdf.
144. "Family Meals," New Jersey Department of Family and Community Health Service, Rutgers Cooperative Extension, accessed June 5, 2013, http://getmovinggethealthynj.rutgers.edu/increase/family+meals/.
145. "8 Reasons to Make Time for Family Dinner," Sarah Klein, September 18, 2009, http://www.health.com/health/article/0,,20410583,00.html.
146. Miriam Weinstein, *The Surprising Power of Family Meals* (Hanover, NH: Steerforth Press, 2005), 207–209.
147. Ibid., 128.

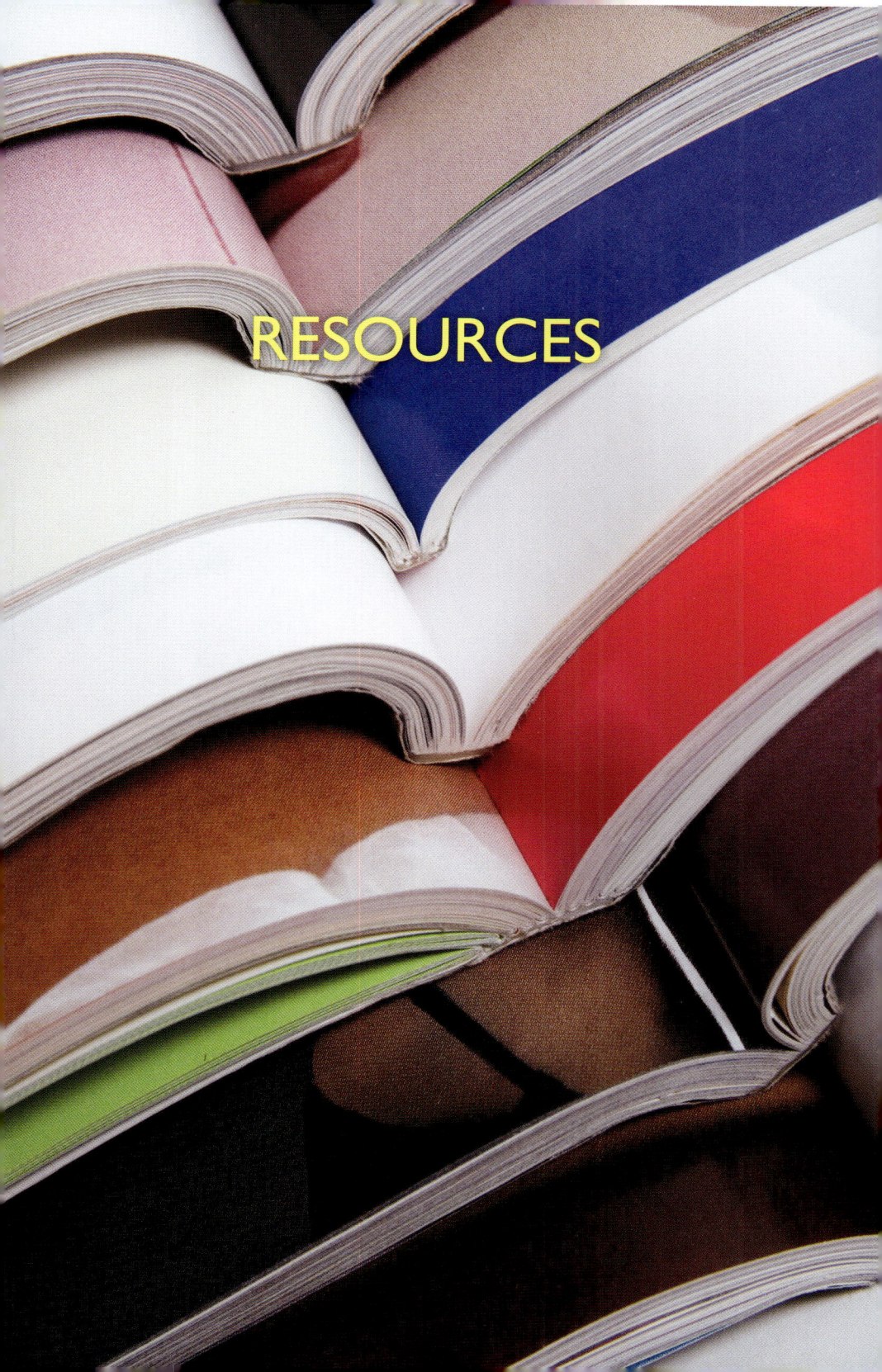
RESOURCES

LEAD YOUR COMMUNITY
TO HEALTHY LIVING

CREATIONHealth.com — Shop online for CREATION Health Seminars, Books, & Resources

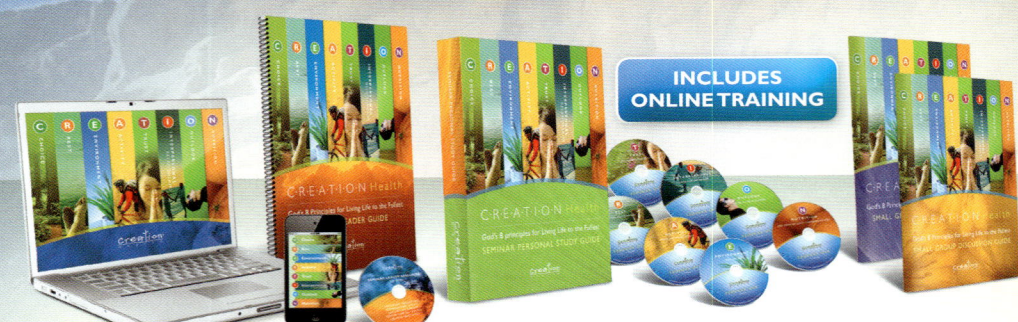

Seminar Leader Kit
Everything a leader needs to conduct this seminar successfully, including key questions to facilitate group discussion and PowerPoint presentations for each of the eight principles.

Participant Guide
A study guide with essential information from each of the eight lessons along with outlines, self assessments, and questions for people to fill-in as they follow along.

Small Group Kit
It's easy to lead a small group using the CREATION Health videos, the Small Group Leaders Guide and the Small Group Discussion Guide.

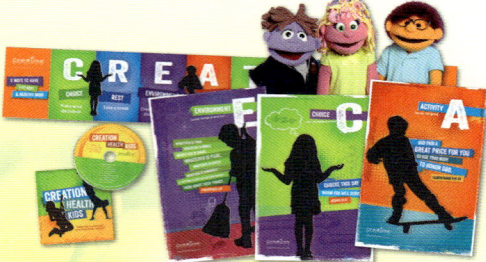

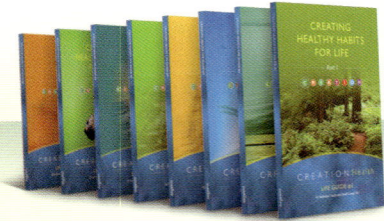

CREATION Kids
CREATION Health Kids can make a big difference in homes, schools and congregations. Lead kids in your community to healthier, happier living.

Life Guide Series
These guides include questions designed to help individuals or small groups study the depths of every principle and learn strategies for integrating them into everyday life.

GUIDES AND ASSESSMENTS

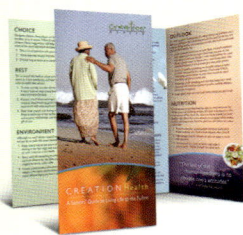

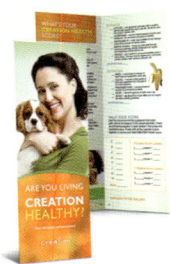

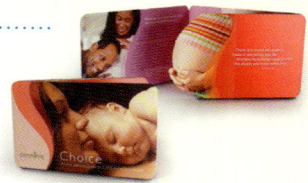

Pregnancy Guides
Expert advice on how to be CREATION Healthy while expecting.

Senior Guide
Share the CREATION Health principles with seniors and help them be healthier and happier as they live life to the fullest.

Self-Assessment
This instrument raises awareness about how CREATION Healthy a person is in each of the eight major areas of wellness.

Pocket Guide
A tool for keeping people committed to living all of the CREATION Health principles daily.

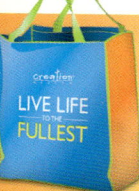

Tote Bag
A convenient way for bringing CREATION Health materials to and from class.

Tumbler
Practice good Nutrition and keep yourself hydrated with a CREATION Health tumbler in an assortment of fun colors.

MARKETING MATERIALS

Postcards, Posters, Stationary, and more
You can effectively advertise and generate community excitement about your CREATION Health seminar with a wide range of available marketing materials such as enticing postcards, flyers, posters, and more.

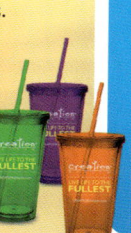

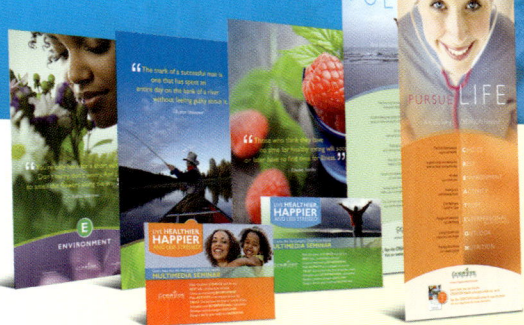

Bible Stories
God is interested in our physical, mental and spiritual well being. Throughout the Bible you can discover the eight principles for full life.

CREATION HEALTH BOOKS

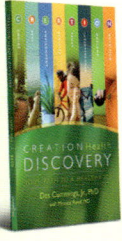

CREATION Health Discovery
Written by Des Cummings, Jr., PhD and Monica Reed, MD, this wonderful companion resource introduces people to the CREATION Health philosophy and lifestyle.

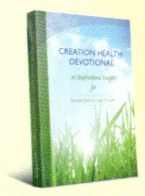

CREATION Health Devotional
In this devotional you will discover stories about experiencing God's grace in the tough times, God's delight in triumphant times, and God's presence in peaceful times.

English: Hardcover
Spanish: Softcover

CREATION HEALTH RESOURCES

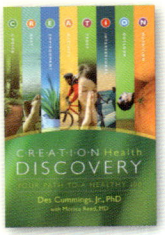

CREATION Health Discovery (Softcover)
CREATION Health Discovery takes the 8 essential principles of CREATION Health and melds them together to form the blueprint for the health we yearn for and the life we are intended to live.

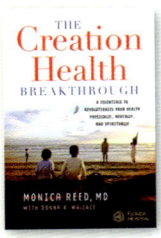

CREATION Health Breakthrough (Hardcover)
Blending science and lifestyle recommendations, Monica Reed, MD, prescribes eight essentials that will help reverse harmful health habits and prevent disease. Discover how intentional choices, rest, environment, activity, trust, relationships, outlook, and nutrition can put a person on the road to wellness. Features a three-day total body rejuvenation therapy and four-phase life transformation plan.

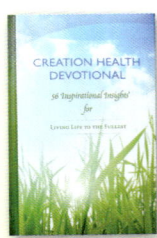

CREATION Health Devotional (English: Hardcover / Spanish: Softcover)
Stories change lives. Stories can inspire health and healing. In this devotional you will discover stories about experiencing God's grace in the tough times, God's delight in triumphant times, and God's presence in peaceful times. Based on the eight timeless principles of wellness: Choice, Rest, Environment, Activity, Trust, Interpersonal relationships, Outlook, Nutrition.

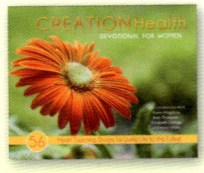

CREATION Health Devotional for Women (English)
Written for women by women, the *CREATION Health Devotional for Women* is based on the principles of whole-person wellness represented in CREATION Health. Spirits will be lifted and lives rejuvenated by the message of each unique chapter. This book is ideal for women's prayer groups, to give as a gift, or just to buy for your own edification and encouragement.

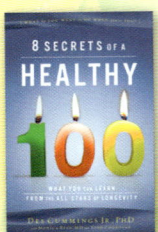

8 Secrets of a Healthy 100 (Softcover)
Can you imagine living to a Healthy 100 years of age? Dr. Des Cummings Jr., explores the principles practiced by the All-stars of Longevity to live longer and more abundantly. Take a journey through the 8 Secrets and you will be inspired to imagine living to a Healthy 100.

CREATION HEALTH RESOURCES

Forgive To Live (English: Hardcover / Spanish: Softcover)

In *Forgive to Live* Dr. Tibbits presents the scientifically proven steps for forgiveness — taken from the first clinical study of its kind conducted by Stanford University and Florida Hospital.

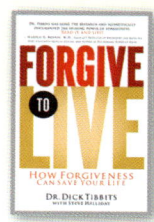

Forgive To Live Workbook (Softcover)

This interactive guide will show you how to forgive — insight by insight, step by step — in a workable plan that can effectively reduce your anger, improve your health, and put you in charge of your life again, no matter how deep your hurts.

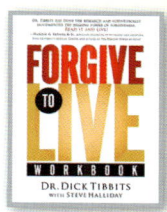

Forgive To Live Devotional (Hardcover)

In his powerful new devotional Dr. Dick Tibbits reveals the secret to forgiveness. This compassionate devotional is a stirring look at the true meaning of forgiveness. Each of the 56 spiritual insights includes motivational Scripture, an inspirational prayer, and two thought-provoking questions. The insights are designed to encourage your journey as you begin to *Forgive to Live*.

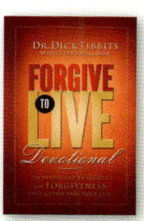

Forgive To Live God's Way (Softcover)

Forgiveness is so important that our very lives depend on it. Churches teach us that we should forgive, but how do you actually learn to forgive? In this spiritual workbook noted author, psychologist, and ordained minister Dr. Dick Tibbits takes you step-by-step through an eight-week forgiveness format that is easy to understand and follow.

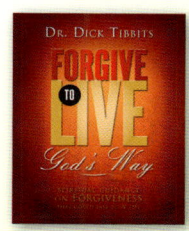

Forgive To Live Leader's Guide

Perfect for your community, church, small group or other settings.
The Forgive to Live Leader's Guide Includes:

- 8 Weeks of pre-designed PowerPoint™ presentations.
- Professionally designed customizable marketing materials and group handouts on CD-Rom.
- Training directly from author of Forgive to Live Dr. Dick Tibbits across 6 audio CDs.
- Media coverage DVD.
- CD-Rom containing all files in digital format for easy home or professional printing.
- A copy of the first study of its kind conducted by Stanford University and Florida Hospital showing a link between decreased blood pressure and forgiveness.

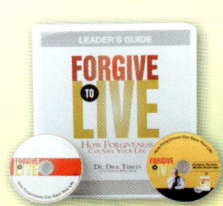

CREATION HEALTH RESOURCES

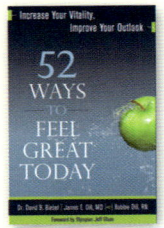

52 Ways to Feel Great Today (Softcover)

Wouldn't you love to feel great today? Changing your outlook and injecting energy into your day often begins with small steps. In *52 Ways to Feel Great Today*, you'll discover an abundance of simple, inexpensive, fun things you can do to make a big difference in how you feel today and every day. Tight on time? No problem. Each chapter is written as a short, easy-to-implement idea. Every idea is supported by at least one true story showing how helpful implementing the idea has proven to someone a lot like you. The stories are also included to encourage you to be as inventive, imaginative, playful, creative, or adventuresome as you can.

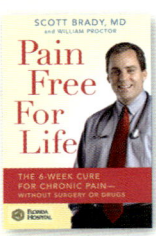

Pain Free For Life (Hardcover)

In *Pain Free For Life*, Scott C. Brady, MD, – founder of Florida Hospital's Brady Institute for Health – shares for the first time with the general public his dramatically successful solution for chronic back pain, Fibromyalgia, chronic headaches, Irritable bowel syndrome and other "impossible to cure" pains. Dr. Brady leads pain-racked readers to a pain-free life using powerful mind-body-spirit strategies used at the Brady Institute – where more than 80 percent of his chronic-pain patients have achieved 80-100 percent pain relief within weeks.

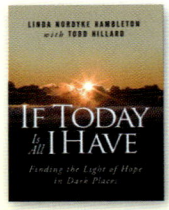

If Today Is All I Have (Softcover)

At its heart, Linda's captivating account chronicles the struggle to reconcile her three dreams of experiencing life as a "normal woman" with the tough realities of her medical condition. Her journey is punctuated with insights that are at times humorous, painful, provocative, and life-affirming.

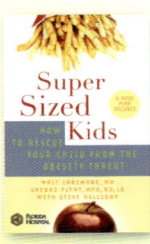

SuperSized Kids (Hardcover)

In *SuperSized Kids*, Walt Larimore, MD, and Sherri Flynt, MPH, RD, LD, show how the mushrooming childhood obesity epidemic is destroying children's lives, draining family resources, and pushing America dangerously close to a total healthcare collapse – while also explaining, step by step, how parents can work to avert the coming crisis by taking control of the weight challenges facing every member of their family.

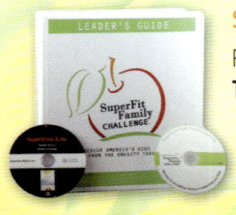

SuperFit Family Challenge – Leader's Guide

Perfect for your community, church, small group or other settings.
The SuperFit Family Challenge Leader's Guide Includes:
- 8 Weeks of pre-designed PowerPoint™ presentations.
- Professionally designed marketing materials and group handouts from direct mailers to reading guides.
- Training directly from Author Sherri Flynt, MPH, RD, LD, across 6 audio CDs.
- Media coverage and FAQ on DVD.

LIVE YOUR LIFE TO THE FULLEST

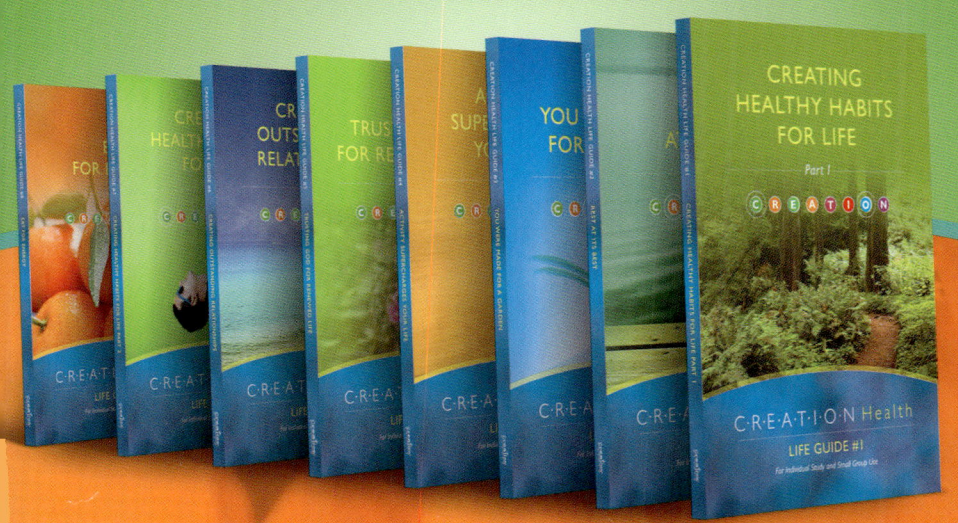

C·R·E·A·T·I·O·N Health

LIFE GUIDE SERIES

8 Guides. 8 Principles. One Powerful Message.
Packed with fresh insights on abundant living.
For Individual Study and Small Group Use.

Perfect for churches, schools, universities, and faith-based businesses.

IMAGINE...

A body that is healthy and strong,
A spirit that is vibrant and refreshed,
A life that glorifies God,
Imagine living to a **Healthy 100**.

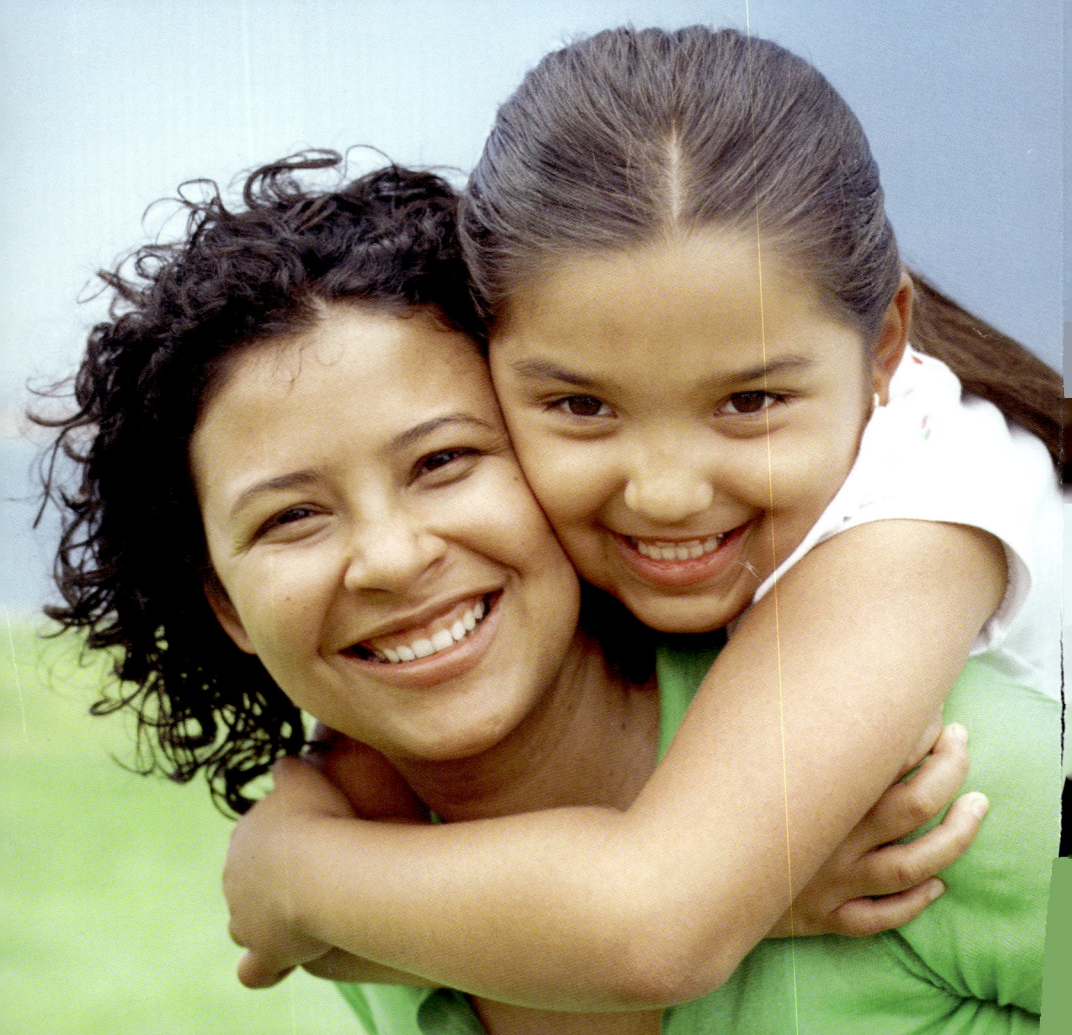